Total Knockout Fitness

Martin McKenzie

Stefanie Kirchner

Human Kinetics

Library of Congress Cataloging-in-Publication Data

McKenzie, Martin.
  Total knockout fitness / Martin McKenzie, Stefanie Kirchner.
      pages cm
  1. Boxing--Training. 2. Physical fitness. I. Title.
  GV1137.6.M36 2014
  796.83--dc23

                                    2013013815

ISBN-10: 0-7360-9434-2 (print)
ISBN-13: 978-0-7360-9434-4 (print)

The web addresses cited in this text were current as of October 2013, unless otherwise noted.

Acquisitions Editor: Justin Klug; **Developmental Editor:** Laura Pulliam; **Assistant Editor:** Elizabeth Evans; **Copyeditor:** Patsy Fortney; **Graphic Designer:** Nancy Rasmus; **Graphic Artist:** Tara Welsch; **Cover Designer:** Keith Blomberg; **DVD Face Designer:** Susan Rothermel Allen; **DVD Producer:** Doug Fink; **Video Production Coordinator:** Amy Rose; **Photograph (cover):** SuperStock/age fotostock; **Photographs (interior):** Michael Yates/Michael Yates Photography, unless otherwise noted; figures 1.1, 1.6 © CIMAC Martial Arts; figures 1.2, 1.4, 1.5 © LE Bolmeer; figure 1.3 © Martin McKenzie; **Visual Production Assistant:** Joyce Brumfield; **Photo Production Manager:** Jason Allen; **Printer:** Versa Press

We thank Solar Studio in Glendale, CA, for assistance in providing the location for the photo shoot for this book.

Human Kinetics books are available at special discounts for bulk purchase. Special editions or book excerpts can also be created to specification. For details, contact the Special Sales Manager at Human Kinetics.

The contents of this DVD are licensed for private home use and traditional, face-to-face classroom instruction only. For public performance licensing, please contact a sales representative at **www.HumanKinetics.com/SalesRepresentatives**.

Printed in the United States of America   10   9   8   7   6   5   4   3   2   1

The paper in this book is certified under a sustainable forestry program.

Human Kinetics
Website: www.HumanKinetics.com

United States: Human Kinetics
P.O. Box 5076
Champaign, IL 61825-5076
800-747-4457
e-mail: humank@hkusa.com

Canada: Human Kinetics
475 Devonshire Road Unit 100
Windsor, ON N8Y 2L5
800-465-7301 (in Canada only)
e-mail: info@hkcanada.com

Europe: Human Kinetics
107 Bradford Road
Stanningley
Leeds LS28 6AT, United Kingdom
+44 (0) 113 255 5665
e-mail: hk@hkeurope.com

Australia: Human Kinetics
57A Price Avenue
Lower Mitcham, South Australia 5062
08 8372 0999
e-mail: info@hkaustralia.com

New Zealand: Human Kinetics
P.O. Box 80
Torrens Park, South Australia 5062
0800 222 062
e-mail: info@hknewzealand.com

E5150

To Eliahs and Samuel and to Joseph and Zachariahs

Contents

Acknowledgments

Special thanks to Stuart Mourant, head of research for Fight Fit Training and Development Ltd., for his invaluable contributions to this book and DVD. Thanks to the team at Human Kinetics, especially Peter Murphy, Laura Pulliam, Doug Fink, and Justin Klug, for their support and expertise throughout this journey. Thanks to some of our clients, who inspired us to write this book: David Harriott, Lloyd Sterling, Jeremey Greenhalgh, Stuart Ford, and Huw Jenkins. Special thanks also to our families for their continued support.

Introduction

This book takes you on an inspiring journey in achieving your health and fitness goals. The calorie-busting Total Knockout Fitness routine is a unique fitness boxing programme that has been enjoyed by boxing champions, elite athletes, celebrities, fitness instructors, fitness enthusiasts and business professionals all over the world.

All those who have enjoyed the Fight Fit training systems have been eagerly awaiting this inspiring mix of fitness boxing workouts with head-turning skipping techniques. A unique food and lifestyle programme supports the Total Knockout Fitness journey to a fitter, stronger body. The step-by-step nutrition and workout programmes will help you in the following ways:

- ✔ Boost your cardiorespiratory fitness and endurance.
- ✔ Burn more calories in a shorter time.
- ✔ Reduce your stress levels.
- ✔ Improve your strength and power.
- ✔ Shape your upper and lower body.
- ✔ Release frustrations.

The chapters feature new, simple ways to work out and provide a huge variety of boxing and total-body training skills and drills to get you into tip-top shape. In addition, to give you that extra visual support on your journey to a knockout physique, some of the workouts you will get to know throughout this book are included on the enclosed DVD.

Whether you enjoy staying fit or are just starting to get into fitness, boxing is a great tool for shaping up and improving your fitness level. It integrates a balance of aerobic and anaerobic fitness, which makes it one of the best ways to get fit, burn calories, increase muscular endurance and improve cardiorespiratory fitness. Using some simple tips to get your mind focused, you can achieve your fitness and weight goals quickly and enjoy the long-term benefits of improved mood, increased energy, improved reaction time and better reflexes.

Whether you are a novice or have done boxing for many years, this book provides unique strategies and breakthrough perspectives on boxing and fitness with new exercises and programmes, ways to maximise focus, and nutrition programmes. Before you get started, make sure you have loose-fitting clothes that allow for ease of movement. A track suit or T-shirt and shorts with well-fitting trainers (sport shoes) will do the trick. To browse our range of workout outfits and learn more tips and tricks, go to www.totalknockoutfitness.com.

And now, let the journey to the healthier, fitter and stronger you begin!

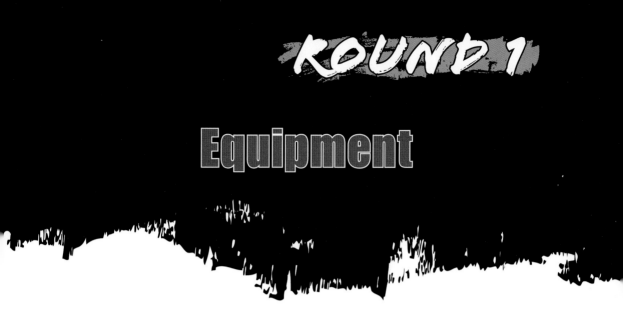

ROUND 1

Equipment

The Total Knockout Fitness programme is a relatively inexpensive exercise programme, at least when you are starting out. The basic boxing equipment you need to get started should last, as long as it is of good quality and suits your needs and requirements. To that you need only add a lot of motivation and determination to make a change in your fitness, health and lifestyle. Your start-up equipment package will consist of gloves, hand wraps, skipping ropes and focus pads; these will give you a sound base to work from. As you go along, punch bags will help you practise more advanced techniques; these include heavy bags, speed bags, floor-to-ceiling bags and standing bags.

Before we go into detail about each piece of equipment, keep in mind that buying good-quality boxing equipment is essential, and such equipment can be had for a reasonable price. These days, you will find the biggest selection online. Type *boxing equipment* into your search engine and compare prices and quality; then make your informed decision.

Always check your workout bag to make sure you have everything you need for your workout ready before you get started. Having to stop your workout to search for a bottle of water, for instance, can be distracting.

Your Total Knockout Fitness Workout Checklist

Before you start your Total Knockout Fitness workout, in the gym, at home or in the park, make sure to pack your bag with some essentials to make your workout more enjoyable. Along with your choice of boxing gloves, bring along the following items:

> Large water bottle (Staying hydrated is crucial for any workout because it keeps your body energised and allows you to work out for longer periods of time.)
> Record book (to monitor your progress throughout your training)
> Waterproof top and tracksuit bottoms (If you work out outside, this is a plus in case of rain or—if you venture out on the coldest winter days—snow!)
> Skipping rope (for your warm-ups and speed-focused training)
> Petroleum jelly (Put some over your eyebrows to stop sweat from running into your eyes.)
> Hand wraps (Make sure you wash your wraps frequently.)

Boxing Gloves

Boxing gloves are cushioned gloves used in boxing-related workouts such as shadowboxing, punch bag routines and working with a partner on focus pads. They come in a variety of styles, but two primary styles are used in the Total Knockout Fitness programme: fitness gloves and bag gloves.

Fitness Gloves

Fitness gloves, as shown in figure 1.1, are for light use, mostly in boxing for fitness and kickboxing aerobics classes, as well as shadowboxing workouts and some light bag work. With the ever-growing popularity of boxing for fitness programmes, more boxing equipment manufacturers are producing this type of glove. They are easy to put on because they don't have any laces and are relatively inexpensive. They range from 12 to 16 ounces (0.34 to 0.45 g), depending on hand size. Fitness gloves don't offer the level of protection that bag gloves or sparring and training gloves do, but some people prefer them. The choice is yours.

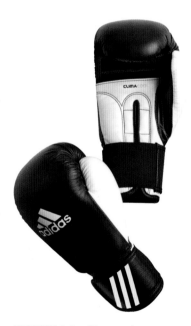

FIGURE 1.1   Fitness gloves

Bag Gloves

Bag gloves, as shown in figure 1.2, are lightweight, easy to carry and affordable. Keep in mind that the lining of bag gloves is not thick enough to provide protection in actual boxing competitions. If you think you will want to take boxing to the next level, consider buying training or sparring gloves, which have greater wrist protection and added stability as a result of thicker padding and lace-ups.

For boxing for fitness, bag gloves are thinner and lighter than conventional boxing gloves. They are mostly used for workouts with a partner, in which one of you holds the focus pads and the other hits them, wearing hand wraps and bag gloves. You can also use gloves to punch bags. Using a punch bag is a fantastic workout, and you can make it as hard or as easy as you want. By varying your speed, duration and intensity, you can customise your workout to your fitness level.

Bag gloves are designed to support and protect your hands and wrists when punching either a focus pad or a punch bag. They are heavier than fitness gloves and offer enhanced wrist support through thicker padding. Like fitness gloves, they often have Velcro closures; however, you can purchase some of the higher-quality versions, which have laces and a protected attached thumb.

Buy quality bag gloves to get the most from your workout and to ensure that you don't have to buy another pair!

They are made of synthetic leather or real leather, while the leather gloves usually provide a longer life. As the name suggests, bag gloves are mainly used for working on punch bags. Bag gloves come in small, medium and large sizes.

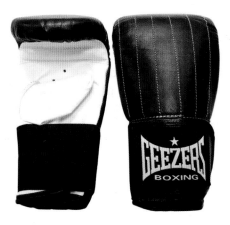

FIGURE 1.2   Bag gloves.

High-quality leather gloves are least likely to let you down. They last longer, don't split easily and don't wear as easily as vinyl gloves do. You can buy bag gloves in small, medium, large and extra large, but make sure to get assistance when you buy your first set. When trying them on, make sure they allow some freedom of movement; if they are too tight, they will restrict the blood flow to your hands and become uncomfortable during your workout. They must also have enough room for your hand wraps, which are discussed in the next section.

If you are really serious about mastering the Total Knockout Fitness routine, you should buy your own gloves; using someone else's can be a very unpleasant experience. You will know what we mean when you take your gloves off after your first really hard, sweat-pouring workout: they won't smell of roses! You can avoid the unpleasant odor of your hard work by using some antibacterial spray on your gloves.

Hand Wraps

Hand wraps should also be on your shopping list. These bandage-like wraps support your wrists, fingers and knuckles and help you avoid injury. They are usually made from 100 percent cotton with a heavy herringbone weave and have a built-in thumb starter-loop design and Velcro closure. They are machine washable as well, so you can keep them clean no matter how much you sweat in the gym.

Hand wraps are an absolute must for avoiding wrist injury by protecting and supporting the tendons, bones and thumbs while punching. They provide the extra support needed when punching thick and dense bags and give your hands extra strength so you don't have to rely on the muscles in your hands and wrists to stay in the same position at the point of impact. Wearing wraps allows you to throw with extra security by keeping your wrists from tilting forwards or backwards when you throw a punch.

The number one rule in boxing for fitness is to keep safe at all times. Because wrapping your hands correctly protects your wrists and hands, always have hand wraps with you and follow the guidelines in this round.

Hand wraps come in a variety of sizes: conventionally, 120 inches and 180 inches (3 m and 4.6 m). Choose the length that you feel most comfortable with and that correlates with the size of your hands. If you have smaller hands, go for 120 inches (3 m); if you have larger hands, opt for 180 inches (4.6 m).

Skipping Rope

You do not need an expensive rope to benefit from skipping. Boxers often use speed skipping ropes because they turn faster than normal ropes, making skipping faster and much harder (which is good for your fitness level!). If you want to increase the intensity of your workouts with advanced skipping techniques, use heavier workout skipping ropes (to build up strength and endurance). Have a look at the various skipping ropes and explore their benefits:

- ✔ *Speed ropes* are lightweight and made for fast jumpers. Woven cloth ropes won't bounce off the ground, but they wear out quickly. Beaded ropes are durable and work great for general skipping routines. PVC speed ropes turn fast and are designed to improve speed.
- ✔ *Leather ropes* are for endurance training and usually allow for speed.
- ✔ *Heavy ropes* improve upper-body and arm strength.

Whatever type of skipping rope you choose, remember to buy the right size. Table 1.1 provides some sizing recommendations.

Table 1.1 Correct Jump Rope Sizes Based on Height

4 ft 10 in. (147 cm)	7 ft jump rope (2 m)
4 ft 11 in. to 5 ft 3 in. (150 to 160 cm)	8 ft jump rope (2.4 m)
5 ft 4 in. to 5 ft 10 in. (163 to 178 cm)	9 ft jump rope (2.7 m)
5 ft 11 in. to 6 ft 6 in. (180 to 198 cm)	10 ft jump rope (3 m)
6 ft 6 in. (198 cm)	11 ft jump rope (3.4 m)

Focus Pads

Focus pads, as shown in figure 1.3, are padded targets attached to a glove and are ideal for improving speed, agility and endurance. Their unique curved shape ensures proper hand positioning, and their precision interior pads guarantee an accurate point of impact. If you use focus pads for your workouts, choose high-quality leather with shock-absorbing, high-density filling to ensure safety and comfort.

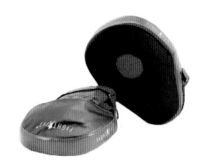

FIGURE 1.3   Focus pads.

Punch Bags

Punch bags are sturdy bags usually affixed to a stand or hung from the ceiling; they are used in boxing training to build speed, power, endurance and precision. They are filled with various materials (e.g., cotton rag, grains, sand), and just like gloves and hand wraps, come in a variety of sizes, usually from 3 to 6 feet (1 to 2 m). For a really effective boxing workout, punch bags are a must. Put on a pair of gloves and start pounding at a punch bag for just two or three minutes. Sweat will show as you burn calories and build strength and speed at the same time. Note that most punch bags need a fitting to be suspended from either the ceiling or the wall, so make sure you consider the space and structure of your workout area before purchasing one.

Many styles of punch bags are available, depending on the type of training you intend to do and your training objectives. To give you an idea of how each bag type affects training, the following sections summarise the most commonly used bags.

Heavy Bag

A heavy bag, as shown in figure 1.4, is used for repeated heavy punching and provides the most resistance as a result of its weight and density. There's no better way to relieve the day's stress than to head to the gym and hit a heavy bag. And you'll be burning calories at the same time! The heavy bag is also a great way to increase the power of your punches, especially when you try to punch through the bag, not just at the bag. You will learn how to do this to maximise your workout later in this book.

You have a few options when it comes to heavy bags, but generally speaking, they weigh about 100 pounds (45 kg) and are filled with hard or soft fill. Hard-filled heavy bags offer more resistance and a stable target because they move around a lot less when you hit them. This allows you to work your arms harder, improve the strength in your forearms and stabilise the muscles in your hands. Heavy bags are made of vinyl, leather or canvas. Leather bags usually last the longest and offer the type of resistance you need when you go through the Total Knockout Fitness programme. Remember: Always wrap your hands when working on heavy bags to protect your hands and wrists from injury.

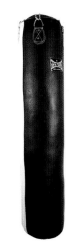

FIGURE 1.4   Heavy bag.

Speed Bag

A speed bag, as shown in figure 1.5, is also known as a speed ball or speed ball bag. It allows you to train rhythm, speed, timing and control over your punches and is designed to improve your eye–hand coordination and help you correctly shift your body weight between feet when performing punches. Slightly pear shaped, the speed bag has an inflatable bladder, similar to the floor-to-ceiling bag, which is discussed next.

The speed bag has a well-sewn leather outer casing that can be inflated to your personal preference. The more inflated it is, the more reactive it is to your punches.

Speed bags come in various sizes, ranging (in inches) from the large 13 × 10 (33 × 25 cm) and 12 × 9 (30 × 23 cm); to the midsized 11 × 8 (28 × 20 cm), 10 × 7 (25 × 18 cm), and 9 × 6 (23 × 15 cm); to the small 8 × 5 (28 × 13 cm), 7 × 4 (18 × 10 cm), and 6 × 4 (15 × 10 cm). Larger bags tend to move more slowly, which means you need to apply more force when punching to keep them moving. Therefore, larger bags are mostly used to work on strength and endurance; and smaller bags, to focus on faster hand speed, timing and coordination.

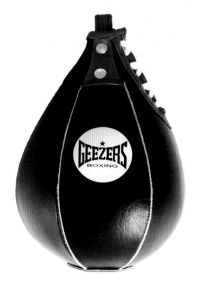

FIGURE 1.5   Speed bag.

Floor-to-Ceiling Bag

A floor-to-ceiling bag, as shown in figure 1.6, is used to enhance reflexes, movement patterns, eye–hand coordination and ultimately speed. It is generally slightly smaller than a soccer ball. A good-quality one is made of leather and well stitched with elastic rubber on either end; it is held by metal clips.

Floor-to-ceiling bags are very similar to speed bags. The main differences lie in the size of the bag and the material they are made from. The cable system of a floor-to-ceiling bag is attached to a clip on the ceiling and a clip on the floor. When you punch a floor-to-ceiling bag, it reacts by swinging towards you, making you move, swerve, dodge and punch, which can vastly improve your coordination and reaction speed.

Many boxing enthusiasts find this type of bag the most fun. With practice, you will learn how to control it, which will pay off by adding to your power and the precision of your punching as well as enhancing your punching-on-the-move skills.

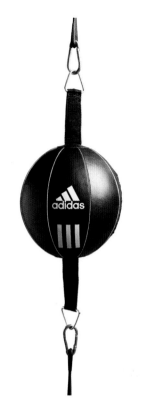

FIGURE 1.6 Floor-to-ceiling bag.

Free-Standing Bag

Free-standing bags are normally used in gyms and health clubs because of building restrictions or lack of suitable support for wall or ceiling fixed bags. Many people opt for this type of bag because it is easy to set up. Although a good free-standing bag might cost a little bit more than other types of punching bags, it may last longer and therefore save you money in the long run. Designs vary, but usually the base is filled with either water or sand; the bag itself is typically made of vinyl or leather. The free-standing bag is used for punching as well as kicking. A good bag will have a wide base, making it more stable. Because it moves during training, you can train for speed, power and strength.

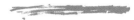

This round familiarised you with the equipment you can use in the Total Knockout Fitness programme: from gloves and hand wraps to skipping ropes and punch bags. Now that you have some insight into equipment, we will move on to testing your fitness level and maximising your diet, and ultimately show you how to use boxing equipment to get a great total-body workout!

ROUND 2

Knowing Your Opponent

Now is probably the best time to let you know that your biggest opponent in boxing for fitness is yourself. For this reason, knowing what you want (e.g., to lose weight, build lean muscle, improve cardiorespiratory fitness or boost your confidence) and where you are at the moment (i.e., your current fitness level) is important to establish before you start the Total Knockout Fitness programme. This applies whether you exercise regularly or are getting back into exercise after a long break (or for the first time).

What's Your Current Fitness Level?

Before you get started with this type of boxing training, you need to find out how fit you really are. Knowing your current fitness level is vital for determining your fitness and weight goals.

The Total Knockout Fitness check your fitness test can be carried out anywhere—the gym, your home, a local park. The exercises outlined in this round test your muscular strength, endurance, power, cardiorespiratory fitness, coordination and balance. Just make sure to rest between tests so you are fully recovered. Each exercise takes 30 to 40 seconds to complete and is followed by a 1-minute rest before moving to the next exercise. Sticking with this format will provide a true evaluation of your progression when you retest yourself, ideally after a week. Testing yourself weekly will reveal your progress and the areas in which you are most improving, as well as those you need to work on. Count and note the number of repetitions you managed to do in the 30 or 40 seconds so you can compare your notes from week to week.

The test includes the following eight exercises.

PRESS-UP

Press-ups exercise the pectoral muscles, the triceps, the anterior deltoids and supporting muscles and the torso and core section as a whole. Press-ups offer a 'push test' of the upper body and stability and functional strength based on your ability to hold the correct postural position throughout. This exercise tests various aspects such as power (when performed as an explosive movement) and strength and endurance (when performed over and over).

To perform the press-up, start in the prone position on your toes and hands with your hands slightly wider than shoulder-width apart and your elbows stiff so they are almost locked. Engage the chest muscles; pull the belly button in towards the spine and squeeze the glutes to stabilise the core. Hips and shoulders are in line to form a flat back (see figure 2.1a). Inhale as you lower yourself by bending your elbows until your chest almost touches the floor (see figure 2.1b). Always lead with your chest, not with your head. Your neck must stay in line with the rest of your spine. Don't look forwards or down because this puts unnecessary tension on your neck! Continue to engage the muscles of the chest and stabilise the core muscle groups to maintain correct alignment. Come back up by pushing the floor away from you through your palms and squeezing your biceps in towards your chest.

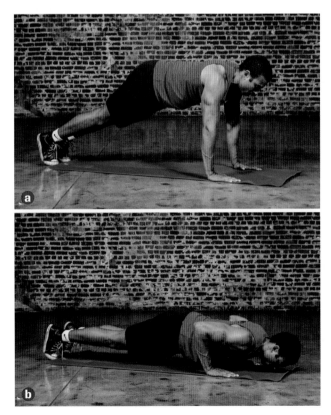

FIGURE 2.1 Press-up.

If the press-up is too difficult, try the box press-up, which requires less strength from the targeted muscles. It is still a good exercise for toning your chest, shoulders arms and provides a great starting platform. To perform the box press-up, place your hands underneath your shoulders with your fingers facing forwards and your knees and feet resting on the floor (see figure 2.2*a*). Make a box shape with your arms, your body, your thighs and the floor. Bend from your elbows and aim to make a right angle with your arms (see figure 2.2*b*). Inhale as you lower your chest towards the floor. You should feel your chest and shoulders working as you push back to your starting position while you exhale.

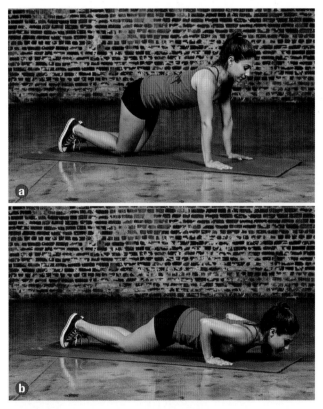

FIGURE 2.2   Box press-up.

BURPEE

The burpee is a total-body exercise involving squat, push, pull and jumping movements. To perform the burpee, begin in a standing position with your feet about shoulder-width apart and squat down placing your hands on the floor (see figure 2.3*a*) in front of you while simultaneously driving your feet back to a press-up position (see figure 2.3*b*). Immediately return your feet towards your chest (see figure 2.3*c*) and drive up as high as possible from the squat position, finishing with a jump and knee tuck in towards the chest (see figure 2.3*d*).

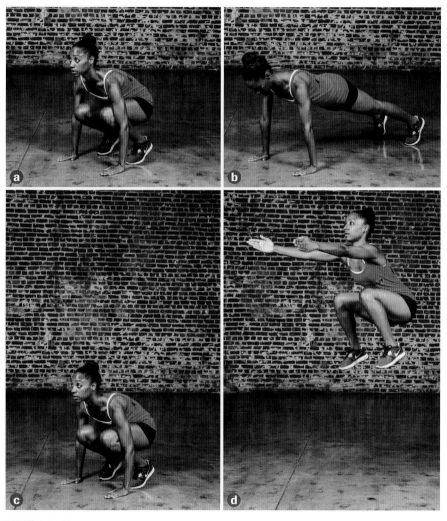

FIGURE 2.3 Burpee.

Because the burpee is made up of a several movements, you can break it down into components to have alternatives that are more suitable for your current level of fitness and ability, as follows:

SQUAT AND THRUST

Begin in a standing position with your feet about shoulder-width apart. Then squat down placing your hands on the floor in front of you while simultaneously driving your feet back to a press-up position.

BRIDGE TO STAND UP

Beginning in the prone starting position for a press-up (see figure 2.4a), pull your knees in towards your chest and drive up to a squat position (see figure 2.4b), finishing by standing upright (see figure 2.4c).

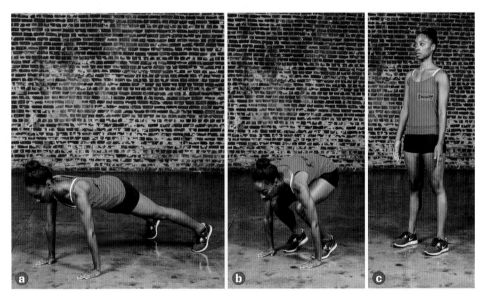

FIGURE 2.4 Bridge to stand up.

SQUAT TO TUCK JUMP

Begin in the squatting position with hands on the floor, knees tucked into the chest and butt into the heels (see figure 2.5a). Push powerfully away from the floor through the legs and up into the air, pushing the chest out while simultaneously driving the knees up towards the chest (see figure 2.5b).

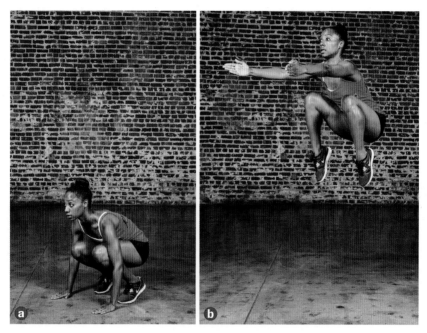

FIGURE 2.5 Squat to tuck jump.

CRUNCH

The crunch, one of the most common abdominal exercises, primarily works the rectus abdominis, also called the 'six-pack muscle'. To perform the crunch, begin lying face up on the floor with about a fist distance between the chin and the chest, knees bent at 90 degrees and feet elevated (see figure 2.6a). Position your fingers at your temples or cross your hands over your chest. The movement begins by curling the shoulders towards the pelvis while maintaining the same distance between the chin and the chest (see figure 2.6b). Focus on a spot on the ceiling while keeping your back flat on the floor throughout the exercise. Eliminating any involvement of the hip flexors makes the crunch an effective isolation exercise for the abdominals. Injury can result from pushing against the head or neck with the hands behind the head, so avoid this type of movement. If this version of the crunch is too difficult, you can perform this exercise with your feet flat on the floor instead.

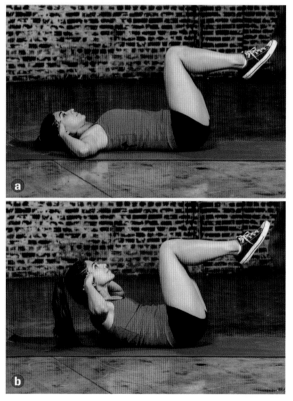

FIGURE 2.6 Crunch.

STAR JUMP

The star jump is predominantly a lower-body and core exercise involving the thighs and butt; however, the star phase does confer some upper-body benefits. To perform the star jump, stand tall with your feet hip-width apart (see figure 2.7a). Inhale and bend your knees to lower your body weight towards the floor so that your butt moves towards your heels and your chest moves towards your knees (see figure 2.7b). Drive up from the feet and throughout the whole body, opening up with the arms and legs in a star shape (see figure 2.7c).

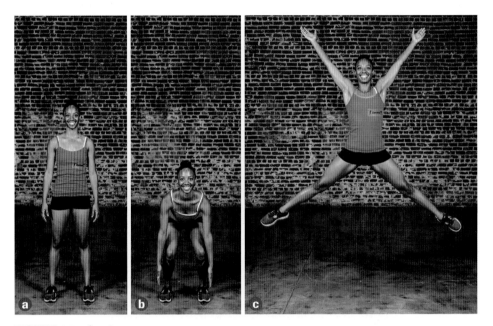

FIGURE 2.7 Star jump.

If the star jump is too difficult, you can perform a jumping jack by standing with your feet together and arms at your sides (see figure 2.8a). Tighten your abdominal muscles to pull your pelvis forwards and take the curve out of your lower back. Bend your knees and jump, moving your feet apart until they are wider than your shoulders (see figure 2.8b). At the same time, raise your arms over your head. You should be on the balls of your feet. Keep your knees bent while you jump again, bringing your feet together and your arms back to your sides. At the end of the movement, your weight should be on your heels.

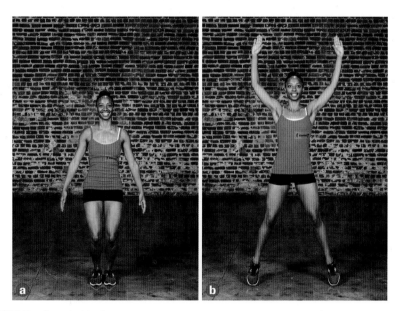

FIGURE 2.8 Jumping jack.

OBLIQUE TWIST

The oblique twist is an abdominal exercise similar to the crunch but with more emphasis on the oblique muscles. When done correctly, oblique twists create a more slender and toned waistline. To perform the oblique twist, begin by lying face up on the floor with about a fist distance between the chin and the chest, knees bent at 90 degrees and feet elevated (see figure 2.9a). The movement begins by curling one of your shoulders towards the pelvis and taking the elbow towards the alternate knee to create a twist movement (see figure 2.9b). Maintain the distance between the chin and the chest by focusing on a spot on the ceiling, and keep the back flat on the floor throughout and to eliminate any involvement of the hip. Place your fingers at your temples or cross your hands over your chest. Do not push against your head or neck with your hands behind your head.

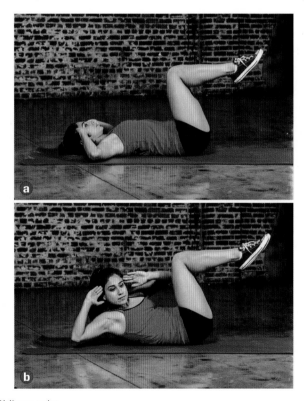

FIGURE 2.9   Oblique twist.

SQUAT JUMP

The squat jump is a compound, total-body exercise that trains primarily the muscles of the thighs (quads, hamstrings), hips and buttocks (glutes) and core (abdominals and deep abdominals). To perform the squat jump, start in an upright stance and midlevel guard (see round 6 for more details on how to perform a midlevel guard) with feet shoulder-width apart. Now step forwards with one foot, turn the rear foot 45 degrees, bend your knees, place your hand in the guard position and tuck your elbows in (see figure 2.10a). Inhale as you squat down by bending at the knees and sticking your butt back as you lower. Keep your head and chest up and your eyes looking forwards, and aim to get your thighs parallel to the floor. Exhale as you drive up through your heels and squeeze your butt (see figure 2.10b). As you leave the floor, rotate so you are in a mirrored stance as you land (see figure 2.10c) and repeat. If the squat jump is too difficult, you can perform squats without the jump.

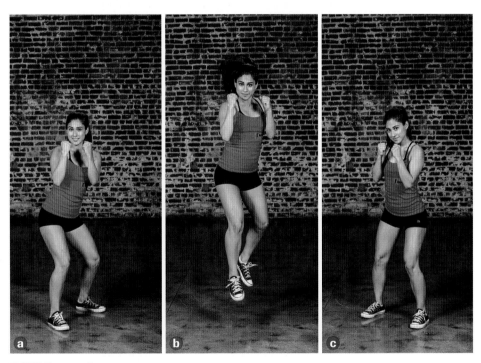

FIGURE 2.10 Squat jump.

DORSAL RAISE

The dorsal raise focuses on the posterior, or back, muscles to strengthen the spinal erectors and transversospinalis group. To perform the dorsal raise, start by lying face down and place your hands beside your head with your fingers touching your temples (see figure 2.11a). Raise your torso and draw your elbows in to your sides, squeezing your shoulder blades together and squeezing your glutes and hamstrings to lift your toes while pushing your hips into the floor (see figure 2.11b). The abdominal muscles will extend or stretch, and the multifidus and spinal erector muscles will tighten in the lumbar region of the back. Contract the abdominal muscles and lower the torso and toes to return to the starting position. If this version is too difficult, you can perform the dorsal raise with your feet on the floor.

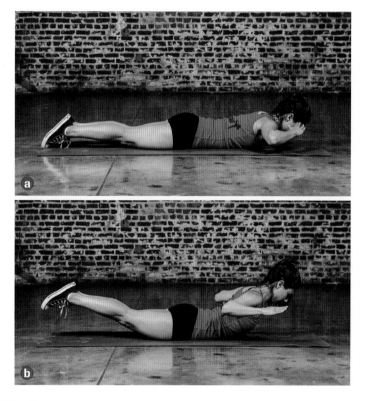

FIGURE 2.11 Dorsal raise.

TOE TOUCH

The toe touch tests flexibility by focusing on the stretching and strengthening of some of the key postural muscles including the erector spinae muscles of the lower back, the multifidus muscles and the hamstrings and glutes. To perform the toe touch, begin in a standing position with the feet close together (see figure 2.12a). Keep the chest elevated and the spine in an extended position while tipping slowly forwards from the hips to stretch the hamstrings and glutes in a hip extension (see figure 2.12b). Other muscles are involved in stabilising and maintaining balance. As you lower yourself down, exhale and let go of any tension. As you slowly rise back up, focus on your lower-back muscles pulling you up while maintaining good postural form and keeping the chest elevated. The degree of knee bend used will change the focus. The straighter the knees are, the more the hamstrings are stretched.

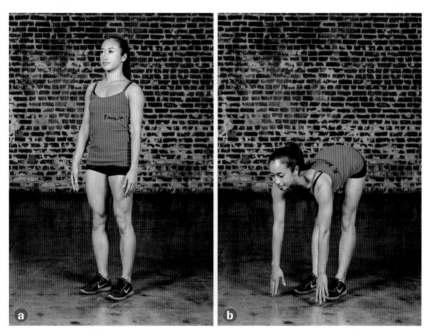

FIGURE 2.12   Toe touch.

Interpreting Your Results

This fitness test is a good starting point for determining your current fitness level and planning a progression to a higher level. Note the reps you managed the first time you performed the test; then, week by week, increase your reps for each exercise until you reach the fitness level you desire. Because the Total Knockout Fitness programme is a progressive training system, you will improve each time you perform an exercise or technique. By consciously engaging a specific muscle, muscle group or movement pattern and identifying key areas of weakness or points of tension, you can strengthen or relax them to increase your fitness level.

Table 2.1 provides a general overview of how to read your results and identify your current fitness level category. Don't be disappointed if your results are low the first time around; the point of this book is to provide ready-made programmes for increasing your fitness level. The purpose of this test is to see where you are at the moment and to help you find the best ways to increase your fitness level.

After assessing your fitness level, your next question is likely: How do I improve? Where do I go from here? The short and only answer to this question is, by giving your body a regular workout and balancing it with a healthy nutrition programme. This book provides great exercises and workout routines that will clearly demonstrate how to improve your fitness level. In round 3 you will find proven nutrition tips that can enhance your general performance and help you look and feel the way you aspire to. You will also learn very simple visualisation techniques that can help you determine and achieve your short- and long-term fitness and health goals.

Table 2.1 Your Fitness Results

| Exercise | FITNESS LEVEL | | |
	Low	Moderate	High
Press-up	0-10	11-15	16+
Burpee	0-10	11-15	16+
Crunch	0-10	11-15	16+
Star jump	0-12	13-15	16+
Oblique twist	0-10	11-15	16+
Squat jump	0-10	11-15	16+
Dorsal raise	0-10	11-15	16+
Toe touch	Can touch the middle of your shins.	Can touch your ankles.	Can touch your toes or the floor.

If you are still deciding how much effort you are willing to put in to improve your fitness level or have not made up your mind about the benefits of becoming fitter, here are 10 reasons for increasing your health and fitness:

1. To reduce risks of coronary heart disease, osteoporosis and many more illnesses you want to avoid
2. To shape up and control your weight
3. To reduce your stress level
4. To have more energy
5. To increase strength and power
6. To sleep better
7. To slow down the ageing process
8. To balance your body and your mind
9. To boost your confidence and brain power
10. To simply feel good about yourself!

This round has been about getting to know your fitness level and ability. You learned how to perform exercises that will indicate how fit your body is and the steps you can take to improve your fitness by performing these tests on a regular basis and increasing your efficiency and endurance to perform more reps step by step, week by week. This round can be a constant companion throughout this programme because you can come back to the test, check your fitness level and find even better ways to become even fitter.

ROUND 3

Tipping the Scales in Your Favour

You have all probably heard the old saying, You are what you eat. To a large extent this is true. What you put into your body determines your concentration level and the way your body and mind performs throughout the day. If you are ingesting high amounts of simple sugar, such as candies, doughnuts, flavoured coffees and soda, which will unavoidably store unwanted fat, your body will burn through the sugar very quickly. This may give you an experience of high activity for a short time, but will almost certainly be followed by a feeling of low energy and lethargy. If you want to give your body maximum benefits through nutrition and lose some weight to achieve the shape you have always wanted, all you need to do is start an exercise routine that you enjoy and make some simple changes to your diet. Bear in mind that whenever you start a new health and weight programme, you should get the all-clear from your doctor or a qualified nutritionist beforehand.

To lose weight efficiently and healthily, you have to know why you gain weight in the first place: when you take in more energy (calories) than your body is capable of burning, you gain weight. The extra calories are stored as fat, and too much fat results in weight gain. If you're also not physically active, you're even more likely to gain weight. Another contributing factor is your metabolism, which regulates how quickly or slowly you burn fat. If you have a fast metabolism, you burn fuel quickly. If you have a slow metabolism, you burn calories from food at a slower rate. The good news is that you can increase your metabolism.

Now is the time to step up to the challenge of managing your weight by making simple changes. This should be part of any programme for getting in shape. All it takes is a commitment and a willingness to slightly

A good diet is key to health, good blood circulation and overall performance at work and in sports.

change your lifestyle and habits. This can be one of the hardest aspects of a programme, but once you make this commitment, you will be on the road to a more active, healthier lifestyle.

So how exactly do you take control of your weight? The good news is that you can manage your weight just as you manage your household or your money. You may think this is easier said than done because you have heard a multitude of theories about how to control weight. The majority of these, though, tend to be fads or crazes. We have discovered through extensive experimentation and research that only a few *really* work and have longevity. The following sections offer tips on how to take control of and manage your weight in a way that has proven to work for a huge number of clients.

Keep a Food Diary

We have worked with many elite athletes who manage their bodies to perform consistently at optimum levels. One of the things that separates them from us 'mere mortals' is that they have been educated and guided by experts to create a balanced diet and a workout programme that suits their body types. This process usually starts with the creation of a food diary. The encouraging news is that anyone can use this tool.

To start your own food diary, for one week, eat the foods and drink the fluids you would usually have and write them *all* down, including the times you consume them. This will be the baseline to work from as you learn how to make positive changes in your diet and lifestyle. See figure 3.1 for a food diary template. Another good idea to make the most of your food diary is to

FIGURE 3.1 Daily Food Diary Template

Name: _____ Date: _____

	Time	What did you eat?	Activities around the time you ate	Your mood	How did you feel?
Breakfast					
Snack					
Lunch					
Snack					
Dinner					
Daily fluid intake					

From McKenzie and Kirchner, 2014, *Total knockout fitness* (Champaign, IL: Human Kinetics).

log your mood and your activities around the times that you eat and how you feel (i.e., did you feel hungry, or did you crave a specific type of food?).

After logging your food intake for one week, identify foods you can substitute with healthier options listed in this round as well as changes in calorie intake to meet your recommended daily intake. A healthy approach is to cut 500 calories from your current diet every week until you reached the recommended intake of about 2,000 calories per day for women and 2,500 per day for men. This recommendation is good as long as your diet is well balanced and you're getting lots of exercise. Especially when following a fitness programme, it is extremely important that you have the necessary fuel for your muscles and are suitably hydrated to be able to tolerate both high- and low-intensity workouts.

> If you are a typical comfort eater, take a minute to think about alternatives that can make you feel at ease without opting for the high-calorie food you usually overindulge in. Choices might include a nice, warm bath, reading your favourite book or magazine or watching a movie you have wanted to see for a long time. The key is to create a pleasant distraction for yourself.

Eat Smart

The next time you go to the store, take a little time to check the ingredients in your favourite foods. You might be surprised at the high levels of sugar, saturated fat and salt. To get the best out of the Total Knockout Fitness programme, you need know how what you eat affects your ability to exercise and the overall quality of your lifestyle.

Checking the ingredients in the foods you buy is a step in avoiding unwanted calories by identifying empty calories and substituting them with tasty foods that give you plenty of energy and comfort. Bad eating habits can lead to a short attention span, high blood pressure, mood swings, heart disease and, in some cases, depression. This is why you should take the time to look at what you are eating and make adjustments—to your meals and snacks.

Having worked with many champions, from boxers to runners, footballers, and track and field stars, we have realised that whether you are at work or play, having the right fuel in your system is critical to your performance. Make simple tweaks to your diet by replacing some of the quick fixes in your daily diet with stable alternatives—for instance, changing black coffees with three sugars per day to herbal teas, fruit juices and water and replacing cream chocolate biscuits and sandwiches with sushi or fruit snacks. By cutting the quick-fix foods out of your diet, you can easily cut down your caloric intake by 1,000, which means you can lose weight even before you start to exercise.

So how do you eat right and use your diet to lose weight and keep it off? Here are a few tips:

Remember the Five-a-Day Rule

It is recommended that you eat five servings of vegetables or fruit a day. Whether fresh, frozen, cooked, raw, tinned or dried, just have your veggies and fruits! Doing this will boost your health and make you look and feel balanced and great. Many of our celebrity clients and sport personalities find that drinking a fresh fruit or vegetable drink is the easiest and quickest way to stay on top of their veggie and fruit intake.

Eat Fish

Eat at least two portions of fish a week, and make one portion an oily fish, such as mackerel, trout or salmon. Fish is really good for your body because the oils in fish are unsaturated fats, maintaining healthy organ function. The high amounts of protein in fish also boost the health of your hair and skin. On top of that, the omega-3 fatty acids found in fish feed your brain and keep your energy levels high.

Replace Saturated Fat

Replace saturated fat with monounsaturated and polyunsaturated fat. Use extra-virgin olive oil (cold pressed) because it is good for the body and helps break down enzymes and assists in breaking down foods. Also, eat fish and nuts.

Make Smart Snack Choices

Avoid calorie-dense or high-sugar snacks such as chips and chocolate bars; instead, opt for slow-releasing sugars that are found in oatmeal, pulses (also known as legumes) and beans. Also, avoid making your snack a meal; keep the size of snacks small. Aim for snacks that are around 150 calories, and don't snack more than twice a day.

Take your time and enjoy every bit of your snack. This will help your body break it down more quickly, won't leave you feeling bloated, will give you a feeling of being full earlier and will give you a break from your day (which for most of us is a good thing).

Add Energy and Health Boosters

Eventually, you will want to integrate some top energy and health boosters into your diet to keep your energy level high throughout the day and maintain good levels of concen-

If you have a busy social life and tend to eat out often, opt for light meals, salads and soup starters and avoid carbohydrate-dense foods because they will only leave you feeling bloated.

tration and focus. Try veggies (especially cauliflower, cabbage and broccoli), cereals, nuts and beans. They are not just great for losing weight; they also boost your immune system. Treat yourself to a selection of slow-release foods such as nuts, including almonds and hazelnuts (which are low in saturated fat), walnuts (which are high in omega-3 fat) and pistachios (which are high in fibre). By integrating foods into your diet that release energy slowly, you provide your body with the sustainable, steady energy supply it needs to function at maximum levels.

Getting a good, balanced source of the vitamins, minerals, protein and nutrients vital to your health will increase your physical and mental productivity, fuel your muscles, aid digestion and provide your body with the essentials for staying healthy.

> Start planning your meals one day in advance. Think about the snacks and meals you will eat the day before and about the layout of your day: when and what you are going to eat? How much preparation time will you have? This simple technique keeps you from waiting until you are hungry to think about food, and then grabbing the nearest thing, which usually means junk.

Eat Metabolism-Boosting Foods

A few simple ways to boost your metabolism are to drink plenty of water and ingest lots of water-based foods such as melon, salad, grapefruit, soup, apples, pears, broccoli and hot peppers. Make sure you have a well-balanced breakfast, and stick to smaller, more frequent meals throughout the day. Don't starve your body because this slows metabolism and is not a healthy approach to losing weight. Skipping healthy meals that give your body what it needs is not a weight-loss strategy; rather, doing so puts your body at risk of losing essential nutrients and having a decreased energy level and slower metabolism. Drinking plenty of water and following a fitness programme enhances your metabolism and results in healthy weight loss.

Limit Processed Foods

Cut down on oily, fatty processed foods (e.g., crisps, fries, chocolate). You probably already know that foods with too much fat and oil are not good for you, but may have never managed to cut down your daily intake of these foods. Well, now it is time to do it!

Most processed foods are low in nutrition and high in calories, which means that they speed up the process of gaining weight while failing to provide your body with the nutrients it requires to function well. Almost all products in supermarkets are processed in one way or another, which means additional ingredients and products have been added to their natural state. Opt for wholemeal flour rather than white, processed flour, which contains fewer minerals and less fibre. Also, avoid fruit juices that have added sugar because they are generally very high in calories and offer less nutritional value than, for example, fresh-pressed juices. Opt for foods without added artificial colours because these have been linked to health problems.

Avoid Drinking Too Much Alcohol

To cut down on the amount of alcohol you drink, a first step is to halve your current intake. Alcohol is generally high in calories and therefore causes your body to gain weight. After drinking alcohol, many people feel the urge to eat food as well, taking in even more calories. Calories are calories, whether your drink them or eat them, so beware of drinking too much alcohol and pay attention to how many calories it adds to your daily intake.

Now that you've learned some key tips on how to eat smarter, it's important to also talk about the quality and frequency of your eating. Any top sportsperson will tell you that eating habits are critical to performance. Now you may not consider yourself a top athlete, but that doesn't mean you can't think like one. The fact is, we can all perform better than we are currently, so what is stopping us from doing so? We are only as good as what we take in whether food or drink or training method. Why not make a change from today and start thinking and eating like a top sportsperson? Come on, give it a go!

As you know, you need a certain amount of calories per day to keep you performing well at work, and obviously, there are various ways to take in those calories. If you took in the recommended number of calories in the form alcohol, for example, your attitude and behavior would likely be poor and your concentration short—not to mention the fact that you might be asked not to come back the next day. This is an extreme example of empty nutrients that don't give your body what it needs to function correctly.

Now consider foods that contain few nutrients yet make you feel full. The question is, full of what? Given the busy lifestyles of today, it is very easy to say that we don't have time to eat well. However, doing so takes a lot less time than you think. With some planning and a bit of forward thinking at the start, eating well will soon become a habit. Planning your diet step by step and getting the body you really want can be easier than you think.

So, what might a typical day look like if you wanted to eat healthier and balance your nutrition? Figure 3.2 provides a complete seven-day nutrition programme that can boost your energy, help you lose or maintain weight and provide all the nutrients your body and brain need to work at their best.

FIGURE 3.2 Seven-Day Healthy Food Programme

	Breakfast	Mid-morning snack	Lunch	Afternoon snack	Dinner
Day 1	One bowl porridge with melon pieces	One handful blueberry and almond mix	One piece salmon (or tofu) with potatoes and salad	One banana plus handful of grapes	One bowl tomato soup with one slice wholemeal bread
Day 2	One piece wholemeal toast with tuna spread	One handful walnut and raisin mix	One plate Caesar salad with hazelnuts and chicken (or vegetarian meat)	One apple and mix of berries in low-fat yoghurt (optional)	One bowl sweet potato and coconut soup
Day 3	One bowl porridge with pineapple or apple	One glass fruit smoothie (kiwi, banana)	One slice fresh tuna (or beans and sweet corn) with egg noodles	One low-sugar cereal bar	One bowl peanut salad with rice noodles
Day 4	One slice wholemeal toast with fruit spread	One glass fruit smoothie (strawberry, blueberry)	Two pieces chicken breast (soya) and bean mix	Carrot and cucumber sticks with yoghurt–garlic dip	One bowl potato, carrot, parsnip soup with curry
Day 5	One bowl of muesli with pumpkin seeds	One satsuma, one kiwi	One piece mackerel (tofu) with spinach and salad	One slice wholemeal toast with Marmite or peanut butter	One plate tomato soya bolognese with egg pasta
Day 6	One bowl Total Knock-out Fitness Muesli (oats with sesame and pumpkin seeds, low-fat Greek yoghurt, taste of honey)	Low-fat cheese with one slice wholemeal toast	Two chicken breast pieces (or vegetarian meat) in coconut sauce with sweet potatoes	One glass fruit smoothie (kiwi, strawberry)	One bowl vegetable soup (carrots, potatoes, onions, avocado)
Day 7	One bowl porridge with banana	One glass fruit smoothie (apple, cherry)	One plate red meat (soy, minced) with spinach and salad	One low-sugar cereal bar	One slice wholemeal bread with avocado spread

Stay Hydrated

Water makes up about 70 percent of your body weight and keeps your body functioning well by flushing out toxins and carrying nutrients to cells. Not drinking enough water can lead to dehydration, which can cause fatigue, lack of concentration and focus and a drop in energy level. By the time you feel thirsty, you are already at least 10 percent dehydrated, so you must make sure to give your body and mind enough water every day! If you and water are not yet best friends, try drinking 250 millilitres (8.5 oz) more than you currently drink per day, every day, until you reach the goal of 2 litres of water per day.

In addition to water, isotonic drinks (water with added glucose, vitamins and minerals) and herbal teas are also options to help you increase your fluid intake. Isotonic drinks replenish minerals you naturally lose when working out while also topping up your energy level. However, I recommend no more than 250 millilitres (8.5 oz) of isotonic drinks per workout per day. This will give you an optimum boost of nutrients your

At least three cups of water are needed to rehydrate your body after every cup of coffee or other caffeinated drink.

Opt for Less Salty Foods

It is advised that you not go over a salt intake of 6 grams a day, which is equal to one teaspoon. Lots of foods and snacks, such as crisps (also called chips) and salted nuts, are very high in salt. These foods don't do your health any favours and avoiding them as much as possible means you are on the way to supporting your body's health. High amounts of salts are found in many common foods such as:

> Canned and packet soups and sauces
> Baked beans and canned vegetables
> Processed foods
> Pizzas and other ready meals
> Bread
> Cereals
> Cakes
> Biscuits

An easy way to reduce your salt intake is to read food labels and choose lower-sodium options. Obviously, at home you can control how much salt you add while cooking and at the table. Consider using pepper, herbs, garlic, spices or lemon juice to add flavour to your food.

body requires during/after your workout. An overload of isotonic drinks means your body won't be able to process the nutrients maximally. Find herbal teas that you enjoy. There is a vast selection of herbal teas and you can surely find a tea that will appeal to your taste buds. Aim to drink one or two cups a day with a little honey to sweeten it. You will see it may help you relax, calm after a stressful day, sleep better and, most importantly, keep you hydrated.

Get Active

For general health purposes, aim for 45 to 60 minutes per workout twice a week. To reach optimum fitness and health, exercise three or four times per week, 60 minutes per workout. Staying active throughout your day is also a great way to keep your body healthy and in shape. This section offers a few tips to go about this.

Turn everyday encounters into opportunities to be more active. For example, take stairs instead of elevators or get off the bus or train a stop earlier and walk the rest of your journey. If you drive to work, park farther away than usual and walk the rest of the way. By the time you get to your destination, you will be feeling alert and focused and will have burned a few calories, too. Remember, early-morning activity can raise your metabolism (the rate at which you burn fat) for up to 18 hours, which means you will be burning more calories for the whole day.

Another key to becoming more active is finding an exercise or workout routine that motivates you and fits with your lifestyle and needs, something you can do consistently on a weekly basis. Ask yourself whether you enjoy training at home, at the gym, alone or in a group environment. If you prefer training on your own, where do you think is the best place to train—in the park, at home or in the gym? People are motivated to exercise by different things. You may get a kick out of working out on the treadmill surrounded by the gym vibe created by other exercise lovers. Or you may just want to clear your mind by working out at home with your favourite music playing in the background. The key is to do what motivates *you*.

This book is all about you. You will find a lot of helpful workout routines and great ideas to make workouts an exciting experience and something you look forward to. They will help you stay engaged, focused and motivated and bring you one step closer to achieving your goals.

Be Motivated

People have many different reasons for wanting to get fit. Perhaps a holiday is coming up and you want to walk along the beach in the sunshine feeling great, or maybe you want to get fit to be in complete control of the way you look and carry yourself. You may be motivated by that sense of achievement you get when you reach the goal of your ideal body, or by the admiration of others about the way you look and how confident you are. Whatever motivates you, focus on it and envision your ideal self.

If the mind can perceive it, you can achieve it. This can be your motto for a fitter you.

Now that you know the health benefits of drinking lots of water, cutting down on your salt intake and staying active and motivated, let's look at some ways of setting realistic health goals, staying focused and motivated and using simple visualisation techniques to bring you one step closer to a healthier you.

Set Realistic Goals

Health and fitness goals can encompass many things. You may want to lose a specific amount of weight or change the way you exercise, eat and drink. By simply noting these goals, you allow yourself to focus on the light at the end of the tunnel. Establish your goals and imagine yourself healthy at your ideal weight. How much weight do you want to lose to fit the picture you created in your mind? How long should you take to lose it the healthy way? What is your healthy weight? Note your goals and keep records on your advancements week by week. If you tried losing weight before but didn't achieve your goal, set a more realistic time frame. Ongoing exercise and good nutrition are the first steps to the new, healthier you. You may need to do some slight tweaking of your lifestyle: If you enjoy high-sugar drinks or fatty foods, simply save them as once-a-week treats! This will really help you reach your goals and stay there.

Think Positively

Thinking positively and reminding yourself about the achievements you are aiming for or have reached already (even if they are only small ones so far) will allow your mind to focus on getting through the ups and downs of your lifestyle changes. Telling yourself how great you feel as soon as you get up in the morning will get your day started right. Even if you find it difficult at times, remind yourself about the things you will have when you stick to a healthy lifestyle: a stronger, fitter body and a more balanced lifestyle with plenty of energy to embrace life as it comes. In the Total Knockout Fitness programme there is no room for negative thoughts; focus your body and mind on the positive to achieve success and stay motivated—all the way! There is no time like now for making better lifestyle choices.

Visualise Your Ideal Self

Think back to a time when you were your ideal weight, and notice how you look and feel. Is there any sound associated with this picture? Notice how others see you at your ideal weight. Good. Now ask yourself what you were doing differently when you were at your ideal weight. Maybe you had a more active lifestyle, or you ate or drank less. Think about it and write it down.

Now go through this simple visualisation process again, but step into the ideal you, making the picture brighter and really feeling yourself as the ideal you. For more information, check out the Total Knockout Fitness website (www.totalknockoutfitness.com) for our weight-loss and perfect visualisation programmes.

Now that you have learned all about healthy, balanced nutrition and simple ways to tweak your lifestyle and eating and drinking habits to achieve a healthier, stronger body that boasts high energy, focus and fitness levels, we will show you how to work out to ensure that your body gets in the shape you have always wanted. In the next round, you will learn how you can start any workout routine the Total Knockout Fitness way.

ROUND 4

Total Knockout Fitness Exercises

This chapter provides you with a comprehensive breakdown of all the Total Knockout Fitness exercises that you will learn and use throughout this programme. You will get to know the purpose of each of the exercises and learn with a step-by-step guidance how to execute the exercises correctly, safely and with the best results for your fitness levels. The exercises are broken down into easy how-to steps and pictures to show you how it's done. So let's get started!

AB CRUNCH

The crunch is one of the most common abdominal exercises and primarily works the rectus abdominis, also called the 'six pack muscle'. To perform the crunch, lie face up on the floor with about a fist's distance between the chin and the chest, knees bent at 90 degrees and feet elevated (see figure 4.1a). Position your fingers at your temples or cross your hands over your chest. The movement begins by curling the shoulders towards the pelvis while maintaining the same distance between the chin and the chest (see figure 4.1b). Focus on a spot on the ceiling while your back stays flat on the floor throughout and to eliminate any involvement of the hip flexors. This makes the crunch an effective isolation exercise for the abdominals. Injury can be caused by pushing against the head or neck with hands behind the head, so avoid this position. If this version of the crunch is too difficult, you can keep your feet flat on the floor during the exercise.

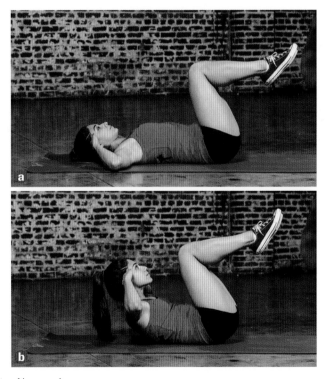

FIGURE 4.1 Ab crunch.

BALANCED LEG SWING

The balanced leg swing focuses on your calves as well as your bottom and thighs, slowly building muscles and shaping you in the right places. Start in a standing position and swing your left leg back (see figure 4.2a) and forth at least as high as your waistline (see figure 4.2b). Repeat with the other leg. As you become more flexible, your legs will swing higher and more fluidly.

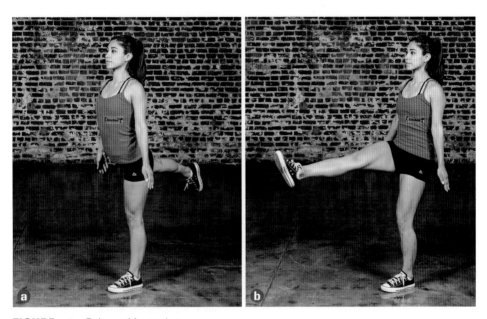

FIGURE 4.2   Balanced leg swing.

BEAR CRAWL

Start in an all-fours position (see figure 4.3a). Raise your knees off the floor to take your body weight onto your palms and toes and crawl forwards (see figure 4.3b). Make sure you stay low to the ground with your shoulders and hips in line and your core braced. Avoid the common mistake of raising your bottom up high in the air and rounding your lower back.

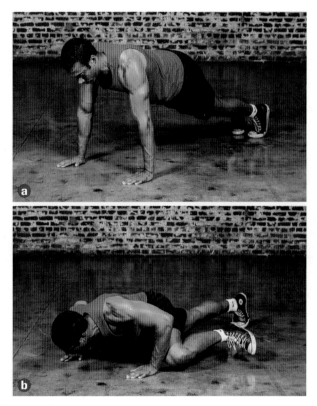

FIGURE 4.3 Bear crawl.

BEND AND FLEX

This exercise is a total-body stretch that also focuses on controlled breathing techniques. Stand with your feet hip-width apart (see figure 4.4*a*) and reach down towards the floor while exhaling (see figure 4.4*b*). Reach the farthest point you can while maintaining correct posture and form.

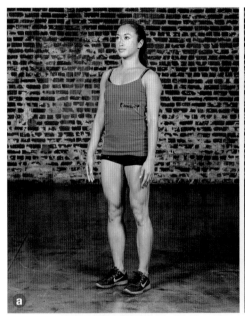 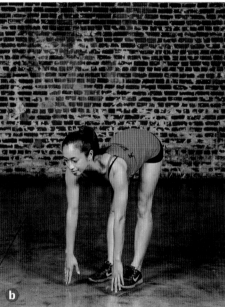

FIGURE 4.4   Bend and flex.

BRIDGE TO PLANK

Get in a press-up position with your body weight distributed through the palms of your hands and toes (see figure 4.5*a*). Starting with your right arm, lower your weight down until you are resting on your elbow (see figure 4.5*b*); follow with the left until you are resting in a plank position with good alignment from shoulders through hips to toes (see figure 4.5*c*).

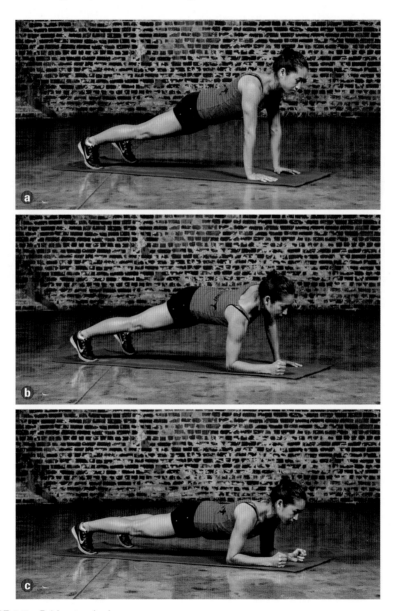

FIGURE 4.5 Bridge to plank.

BURPEE

The burpee is a total-body exercise involving squat, push, pull and jumping movements. To perform the burpee, begin in a standing position with your feet about shoulder-width apart and squat down placing your hands on the floor (see figure 4.6a) in front of you while simultaneously driving your feet back to a press-up position (see figure 4.6b). Immediately return your feet towards your chest (see figure 4.6c) and drive up as high as possible from the squat position, finishing with a jump and knee tuck in towards the chest (see figure 4.6d).

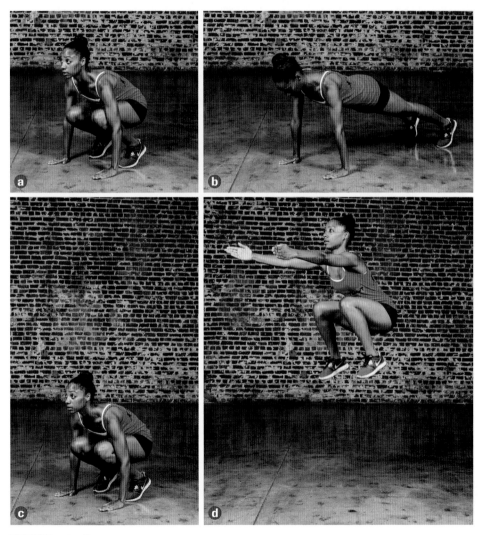

FIGURE 4.6 Burpee.

BUTT KICKBACK

The butt kickback is great for toning bum, hips and thighs. Begin on your hands and knees on the floor with your knees bent at 90 degrees so your thighs are perpendicular to the floor (see figure 4.7a). Keeping your head up, lift your left leg back and up, maintaining your 90-degree knee bend, until your foot is higher than your head or your thigh is horizontally in line with your torso (see figure 4.7b). Squeeze your left gluteus and slowly lower your leg back to the starting position. Perform the same with your right leg, and repeat.

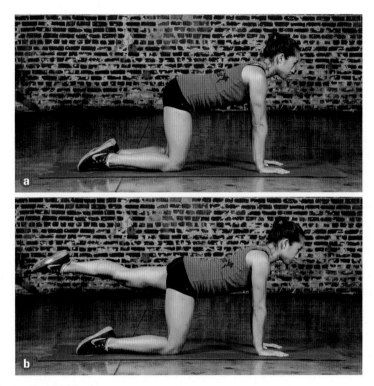

FIGURE 4.7   Butt kickback.

DORSAL RAISE

The dorsal raise focuses on the posterior, or back, muscles to strengthen the spine erectors and transversospinalis group. To perform the dorsal raise, start by lying face down and place your hands to the sides of your head with your fingers touching your temples (see figure 4.8a). Raise your torso and draw your elbows in to your sides squeezing your shoulder blades together and squeezing your glutes and hamstrings to lift your toes while pushing your hips into the floor (see figure 4.8b). The abdominal muscles will extend, or stretch, and the multifidus and spinal erector muscles will tighten in the lumbar region of the back. Contract the abdominal muscles and lower the torso and toes to return to the starting position. If this version is too difficult, you can keep your feet on the floor while performing the dorsal raise.

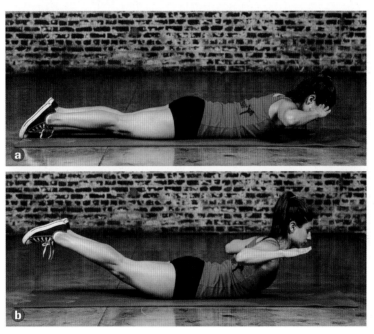

FIGURE 4.8   Dorsal raise.

GLUTE KICK

Glute kicks activate the hamstrings and glutes. This stretch essentially follows the same technique as high-knees running. The only difference is that you keep your thighs perpendicular to the ground while kicking your heels up towards your backside. Stand upright with a slight forward lean, and keep your body aligned with your eyes forward and chin up (see figure 4.9a). Run with arms swinging in a brief motion, exaggerating the height of the knees to bring the thighs parallel to the ground. Kick your heel back until it hits your bottom (see figure 4.9b). Your stride should be short and fast; stay on the balls of your feet and quickly leave the ground each time your foot lands. Repeat quickly on both sides.

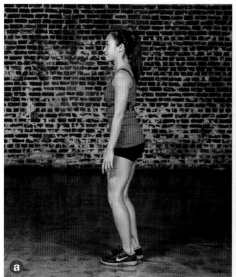 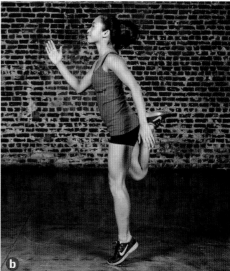

FIGURE 4.9 Glute kick.

HALF BURPEE

Begin by standing up tall with your feet about shoulder-width apart (see figure 4.10a). Squat down placing your hands on the floor in front of you (see figure 4.10b) and drive your feet back to a press-up position (see figure 4.10c). Immediately return your feet towards your chest (see figure 4.10d) and drive up as high as possible from the squat position to land in the starting position (see figure 4.10e).

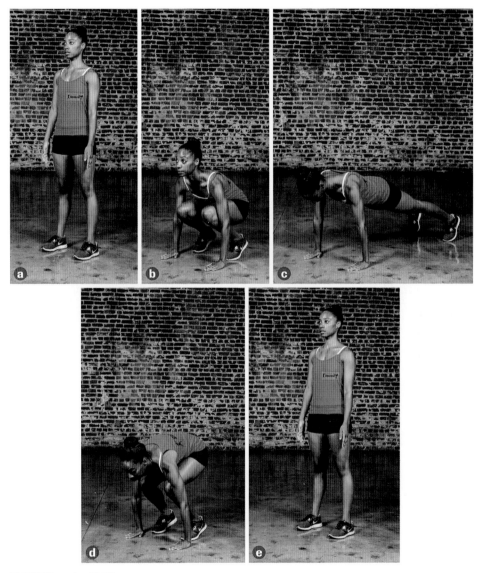

FIGURE 4.10 Half burpee.

HAMSTRING AND CALF STRETCHES

These stretches focus on preparing the muscles for exercise by increasing the range of motion gradually and safely.

1. Sit on the floor with both of your legs straight out in front of you. Bend one of your legs and bring it towards your chest, holding on to your ankle for additional support. Hold for 20 seconds and repeat with the other leg. See figure 4.11 for an example of this stretch.

2. Lie flat on your back, hold one thigh with both hands and bring it towards your chest so that your leg bends. Slowly bring your leg back to a straight position. Hold for 20 seconds and repeat with the other leg. See figure 4.12 for an example of this stretch.

3. Place your palms against a wall and bring one leg back so your heel presses against the floor. The other leg should be positioned in a comfortable, slightly bent position. Keeping your back straight and your heel against the floor, lunge forwards slowly with the front leg until you feel a stretching of the calf muscles of the back leg. Hold for 20 seconds and repeat with the other leg. See figure 4.13 for an example of this stretch.

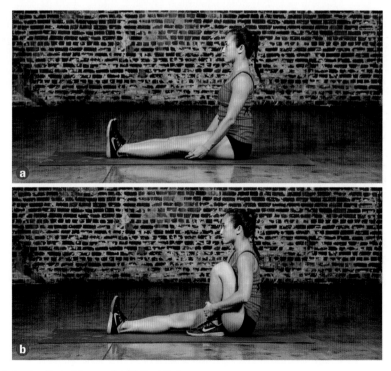

FIGURE 4.11   Hamstring and calf stretch 1.

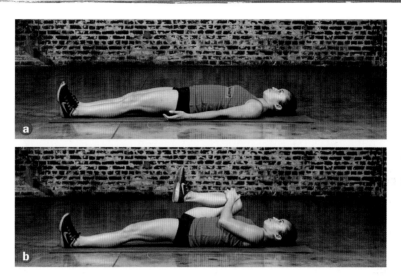

FIGURE 4.12   Hamstring and calf stretch 2.

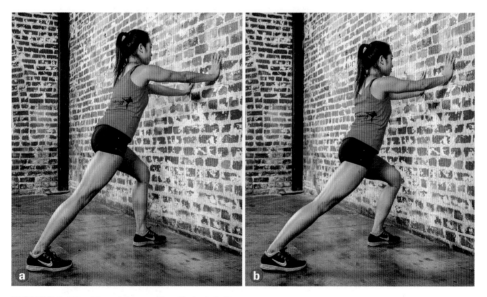

FIGURE 4.13   Hamstring and calf stretch 3.

HAND STRETCHES

A very simple but effective finger and wrist stretch is used in the Total Knock-out Fitness programme to loosen stiff fingers, hands and wrists and help the hands become more flexible so they are faster, stronger and more precise when throwing punches. Practise the following hand stretches daily, and you will feel the benefits very soon.

To perform the wrist stretch, keep the back of the neck and spine lengthened and the rib cage lifted and do the following:

> Start with the right hand and gently extend the fingers back one by one. Repeat on the left hand. See figure 4.14 for an example of this stretch.

> Now take the fingers of your right hand all back at the same time to open your palm, and repeat three times. Repeat on the left hand. See figure 4.15 for an example of this stretch.

> Take your right thumb back towards your wrist. Then bring it forwards, stretching gently and firmly. Repeat on the left hand. See figure 4.16 for an example of this stretch.

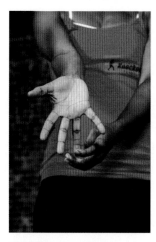

FIGURE 4.14 Hand stretches: extending the fingers back one by one.

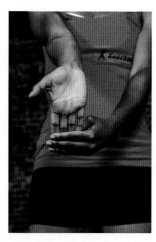

FIGURE 4.15 Hand stretches: extending the fingers back at the same time.

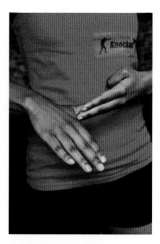

FIGURE 4.16 Hand stretches: stretching the thumb.

> Make a fist with your right hand and slowly open it, stretching your fingers and thumb out as far as you can. Repeat on left hand. See figure 4.17 for an example of this stretch.

> Put your palms together, fingers pointing upwards, as if you were praying. Stretch your fingers and press your palms together strongly. Keep the bases of your palms pressing together as you gradually lower your hands until your lower arms are horizontal. Bring your hands down still further, keeping your fingers and upper palms together. You should feel the stretch on the insides of your fingers and wrists. Hold for a few seconds, and then repeat three times. See figure 4.18 for an example of this stretch.

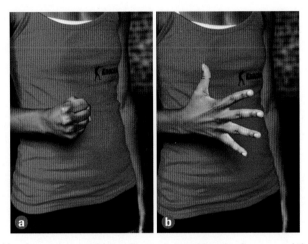

FIGURE 4.17   Hand stretches: making a fist and stretching the fingers and thumb.

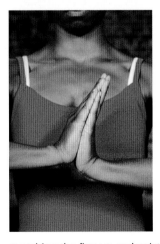

FIGURE 4.18   Hand stretches: stretching the fingers and wrists with the palms together.

HIGH-KNEES RUNNING

High-knees running activates the hip flexors and stretches the glutes. This is a basic form of running except that you bring your knees up higher than normal—ideally beyond your waistline. Stand upright and keep your body aligned with your eyes forward and chin up. Run with arms swinging in a brief motion, exaggerating the height of the knees to bring the thighs parallel to the ground (see figure 4.19). Your stride should be short and fast; stay on the balls of your feet and quickly leave the ground each time your foot lands. Aim to keep your feet moving as fast as possible and your ankles, knees, hips and shoulders facing forwards.

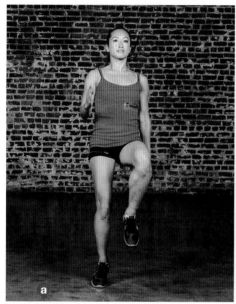 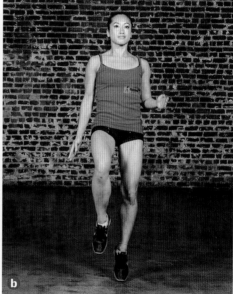

FIGURE 4.19   High-knees running.

HIP FLEXION WITH ROTATION

This exercise increases the range of movement in your hips and shoulders. Stand with your feet just wider than hip-width apart (see figure 4.20a). Tip forwards slowly from the hips, keeping a straight back (see figure 4.20b), and rotate from the hips; now reach your right hand towards the left foot (see figure 4.20c). Repeat on the other leg and reach with your left hand towards your right foot.

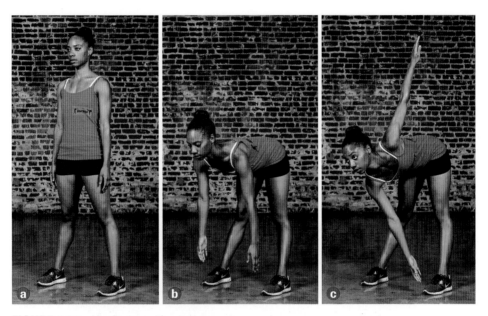

FIGURE 4.20 Hip flexion with rotation.

HIP ROTATION

This exercise improves the flexibility of your hips, thighs and bottom. Begin on all fours (see figure 4.21a). Your shoulders should be in line with your hips; your back, flat; your hands, below your shoulders; and your knees, under your hips. Lift the right leg out to the side and then bring the knees back together (see figure 4.21b). Repeat with the left leg.

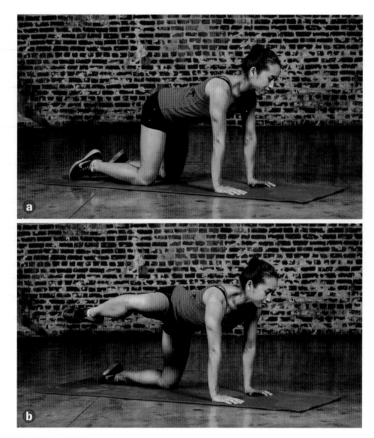

FIGURE 4.21   Hip rotation.

INWARD SHOULDER STRETCH

This exercise stretches the shoulders and hands. Reach the left hand from the small of the back toward the right shoulder blade (see figure 4.22a). Now reach your right hand behind your head and try to touch the left shoulder blade (see figure 4.22b). Hold for 20 seconds and switch arms. The goal of this stretch is to touch the opposite shoulder blade.

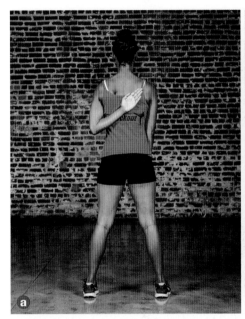 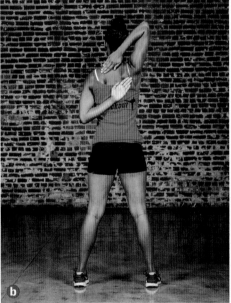

FIGURE 4.22 Inward shoulder stretch.

JOG ON THE SPOT

As the name suggests, this exercise involves simply jogging on the spot for around two minutes to increase your heart rate and warm up your muscles. Be sure to keep your knees soft and land gently on the floor rather than hitting the floor hard, which will increase the risk of knee injury. Allow your arms and shoulders to gently swing by your sides, relaxed. Later, when you have learned the main punches, you can throw punches above your head for a specific amount of time while you jog on the spot to make the most of this exercise and give it a little twist.

JUMPING LUNGE

The jumping lunge is another explosive power movement that develops your primary muscles. Begin by doing a lunge, bringing your back knee to within 5 centimetres (2 in.) of the ground and align your front knee over your foot (see figure 4.23*a*). From the lunge position, jump upwards and drive your arms upwards to increase momentum and explosiveness (see figure 4.23*b*). In midair, switch your legs so that you land with your other leg forwards in a similar alignment and drop down into another lunge. Make your movements explosive, and aim for as much 'air time' as possible.

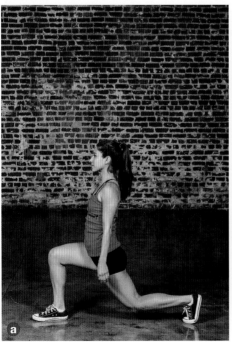 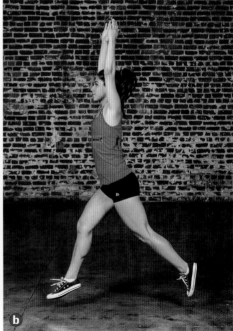

FIGURE 4.23   Jumping lunge.

LATERAL LUNGE

This exercise increases the tone and flexibility of the adductors, or inner thighs. Stand with your feet close together and keep your chest upright, looking forwards (see figure 4.24a). Take a wide step out to the side, keeping your head up and chest upright, and lift your arms until they are parallel to your shoulders or, alternatively, across your chest (see figure 4.24b). Now lower your weight onto your leading leg, keeping your knee in line with your toes (see figure 4.24c).

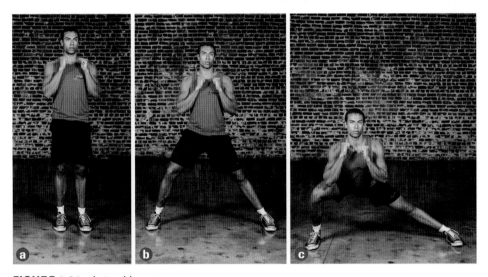

FIGURE 4.24 Lateral lunge.

LOW-INTENSITY SHADOWBOXING

By fixing some tape to a mirror, you can mark some key points such as your central axis and the position of your elbows. Make a cross to mark a specific target such as the centre of your chin to help with your technique.

Adopt the upright stance and midlevel guard position with your feet shoulder-width apart. Take a natural step forwards with the lead foot, keeping the shoulders in line with the toes; turn the rear foot out 45 degrees (this foot position forms a triangle with the backside) and bend your knees. Raise your hands above your head, bring your fingers down and place your thumbs over the outside of your fists. Drop your elbows in to protect your ribs, and hold your fists in line with your jaw, palms facing inwards. Tipping slightly forwards from your hips, place 70 percent of your body weight on the balls of your feet and aim for a specific point directly in front of your chin. Incorporating total-body movement and rotating around your central axis, perform a continuous jab-cross-hook-uppercut combination for five reps. Use a steady pace, without using maximum power, to prepare your muscles and focus your mind for exercise. The purpose of low-intensity shadowboxing is to warm up for the movements to come rather than tire you out before the main session even starts, so keep the intensity low. Concentrate on technique and fluidity rather than speed and power.

LUNGE WALK WITH ROTATION

The lunge walk with rotation is a leg-strengthening exercise with a lot of core and shoulder involvement. This movement strengthens primary muscles such as quads, glutes, hamstrings, obliques and deltoids. If you want to add some weight to this exercise, select an appropriately sized medicine ball or dumbbells. We generally recommend around a 5- or 6-kilogram (11 or 13 lb) ball for men and a 3- or 4-kilogram (7 or 9 lb) ball for women. Start in a standing position (see figure 4.25a). Begin the movement by taking a step forwards and lunging down so that the back knee is just off the ground. The front knee must remain above the front ankle and not deviate too far forwards or to either side. Keeping the upper body vertically aligned and straight, raise your arms out in front of you until your arms are nearly straight (see figure 4.25b). Now rotate your upper body to the front-leg side until your hands are by your front-leg hip (see figure 4.25c). Twist the upper body back to straight, pull the ball or weight back towards you if using weight, stand up over the front leg and then stride forwards into the next step and repeat on the other side.

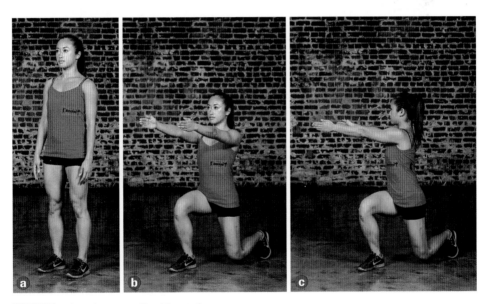

FIGURE 4.25   Lunge walk with rotation.

LYING KNEE TO CHEST

This exercise improves the flexibility of your hamstrings, glutes, lower back and hip flexors. Lie flat on the floor (see figure 4.26a) and bring one leg up towards your chest and grip it with your hands. Pull your leg as close to your chest as you can and feel the stretch through the backside and thigh of that leg (see figure 4.26b). Repeat on the other leg.

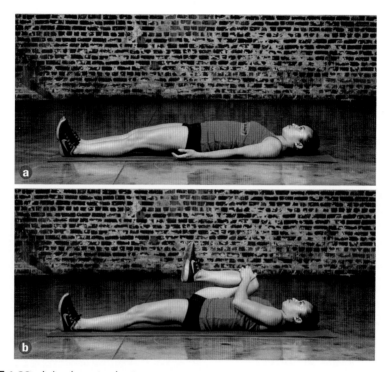

FIGURE 4.26   Lying knee to chest.

MULTIDIRECTIONAL SQUAT THRUST

Start with your hands and feet on the floor in the press-up position and your back parallel to the floor (see figure 4.27a). Keep your hands still and jump your feet forwards as far as you can towards your elbows (see figure 4.27b); then jump your feet back again so your legs are outstretched over to the left (see figure 4.27c). Jump your feet forwards again (see figure 4.27d) and then outstretch them to the right. Repeat for the suggested time.

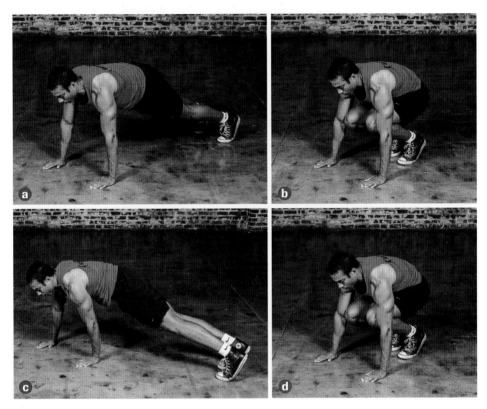

FIGURE 4.27 Multidirectional squat thrust.

OUTWARD SHOULDER STRETCH

This exercise stretches the shoulders and triceps and releases tension in the neck and back area. Reach your hand behind your head (see figure 4.28) and try to touch the opposite shoulder blade. Hold and repeat with the other arm.

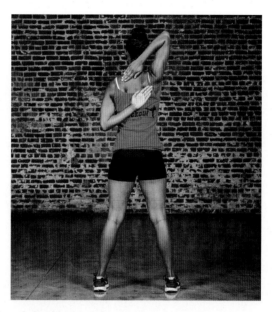

FIGURE 4.28   Outward shoulder stretch.

OVER THE FENCE

Over the fence focuses on your leg muscles, strengthening them to prepare them for your main session. Face in the opposite direction to the way you want to move. Raise your left knee as high as possible (see figure 4.29a) and step back as if you were trying to walk backwards and step over a fence (see figure 4.29b). When stepping over the imaginary fence, keep your upper body straight and your shoulders relaxed. Repeat with the right leg and continue, alternating legs.

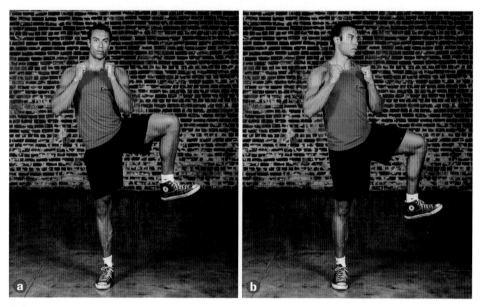

FIGURE 4.29 Over the fence.

PENDULUM LUNGE

Start with feet together (see figure 4.30a) and lunge forwards with your right foot keeping your left foot in the starting position (see figure 4.30b). Now reverse the movement through the full range ending with the right foot in a rear lunge position (see figure 4.30c). Return to the starting position and change legs.

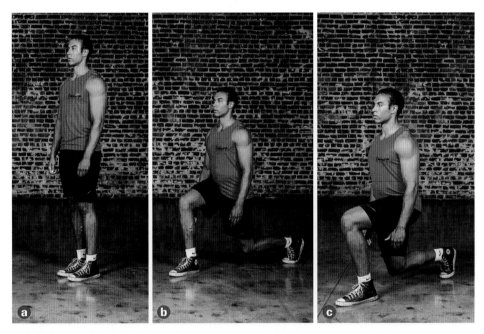

FIGURE 4.30 Pendulum lunge.

PHA CIRCUIT

This specialised training, called peripheral heart action (PHA) training, involves alternating upper- and lower-body resistance exercises and interspersing them with short bursts of cardiorespiratory activity. When alternating between upper- and lower-body exercises, the heart has to work hard to pump blood from one area to the other, making the cardiovascular system work harder and thereby become stronger. This is just what you need to boost your cardiorespiratory fitness.

HIGH-KNEE RAISE WITH LATERAL LEAP

Begin by running on the spot and pumping your arms. With each step, lift your knees to a 90-degree angle or higher (see figure 4.31*a*). After you have completed 10 knee raises (5 with each leg), place both feet together on the floor, load your legs with your body weight and leap to the left (see figure 4.31*b*). Follow this with 10 more high-knee raise (5 with each leg) and leap to the right. Continue for the required time period.

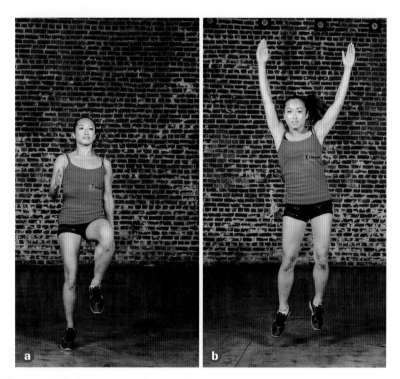

FIGURE 4.31   High-knee raise with lateral leap.

BRIDGE TO PLANK

Get in a press-up position with your body weight distributed through the palms of your hands and toes (see figure 4.32*a*). Starting with the left arm, lower your weight until you are resting on your elbow (see figure 4.32*b*) and follow with the right arm until you are resting in a plank position with good alignment from shoulders through hips to toes (see figure 4.32*c*). Pause momentarily to ensure correct posture (pause longer to build muscle strength or faster to build endurance) and then reverse the movement to return to the bridge position as at the start.

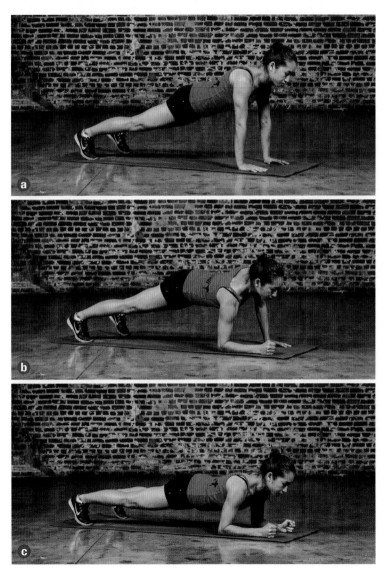

FIGURE 4.32   Bridge to plank.

PLANK

The plank is great for toning your core muscles. Position yourself on your elbows and knees, straighten your legs and raise your body to create a straight line from your head to your toes (see figure 4.33). Be careful not to raise your hips or let them sag, and avoid tensing your neck. Hold this position for as long as you can maintain perfect form, extending the time as you get stronger.

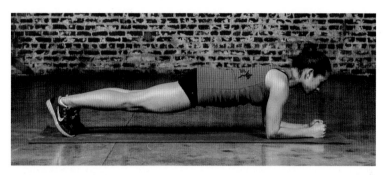

FIGURE 4.33   Plank.

PLANK WITH ALTERNATE LEG RAISE

The plank with alternate leg raise is great for toning your core muscles, glutes and thighs. Position yourself on your elbows and knees, straighten your legs and raise your body to create a straight line from your head to your toes (see figure 4.34a). Be careful not to raise your hips or let them sag, and avoid tensing your neck. Hold this position for a moment to steady yourself; then, squeezing the butt, raise your right leg about 15 centimetres (6 in.) from the floor (see figure 4.34b). Pause for three seconds, lower and repeat with the opposite leg.

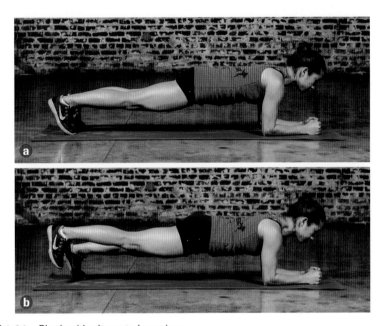

FIGURE 4.34 Plank with alternate leg raise.

PLANK WITH ROTATIONAL REACH

This exercise increases flexibility in your shoulders and spine. Start in a press-up position, maintaining good alignment through the shoulders and hips and with your body weight resting on your toes (see figure 4.35a). Brace your core and lift one hand from the floor while supporting your body weight with the other. Twist your torso and reach your free hand directly behind your supporting arm as far as possible while maintaining good form (see figure 4.35b). Return and repeat on the opposite side.

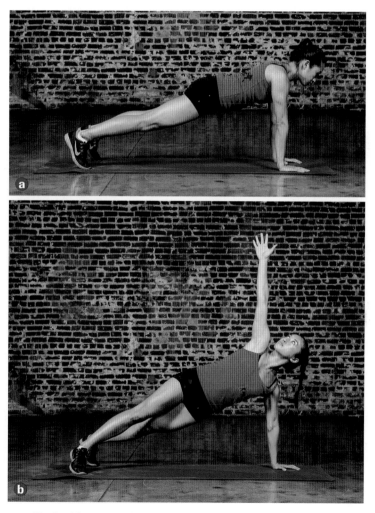

FIGURE 4.35 Plank with rotational reach.

PRESS-UP

Lie chest down with your hands at shoulder level, your palms flat on the floor and slightly more than shoulder-width apart and your feet together and parallel to each other (see figure 4.36a). Look forwards rather than down at the floor. The first contact you make with the floor with any part of your face should be with your chin, not your nose. Keep your legs straight and your toes tucked under your feet.

Straighten your arms as you push your body up off the floor (see figure 4.36b). Keep your palms fixed and your body straight. Try not to arch your upper or lower back as you push up. Exhale as your arms straighten out and pause for a moment. Lower your body slowly until your chest touches the floor by bending your arms and keeping your palms fixed. Keep your body straight and feet together and try not to bend your back. Keep your knees off the floor, and inhale as you bend your arms. Pause for a moment. Begin straightening your arms for a second press-up.

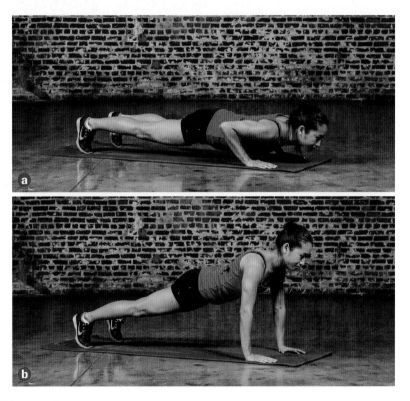

FIGURE 4.36   Press-up.

You can also perform a two-speed press-up, where you perform a normal press-up, but lower yourself more slowly than usual (count for three full seconds) and press up fast (within one second you should be in the starting position again). You can choose from three press-up levels, depending on your ability level: (1) the box press-up, in which your knees are on the floor and your feet are at right angles to your knees; (2) the box press-up in which your knees are on the floor and your feet are lifted at 45-degree angles; or (3) a press-up in which your legs are fully extended and you rest on your toes.

In addition, a simple alternative to the press-up is the sky dive. This exercise builds biceps, triceps and chest muscles, thereby adding extra power to your punches. To perform the sky dive, lie flat on the floor, face down, with your arms by your sides. Gently and slowly raise your chest off the floor until you can feel your lower back muscles start to work; simultaneously raise your legs off the floor as high as you can, turn your arms up, palms facing upwards, and with your thumbs farthest from your body, point to the ceiling. When fully extended, clench your bottom.

If you are already completely confident with the normal press-up routine, you may want to try the advanced version. When performing the press-up, put your hands in different positions (e.g., don't keep them in line, put one hand slightly farther down and the other hand slightly farther up than in the usual press-up position). Repeat on each side. This exercise is also very good for posture, working muscle parts that are not worked in a normal press-up exercise.

PRESS-UP AND HOLD

The press-up and hold is great for toning chest, arms, shoulders and core. Adopt the press-up position making sure that your shoulders and hips are in line throughout (see figure 4.37a). Inhale and lower the chest towards the floor; at the lowest point, pause for three to five seconds (see figure 4.37b) and brace your core as you exhale and drive up through the palms as if to push the floor away (see figure 4.37c).

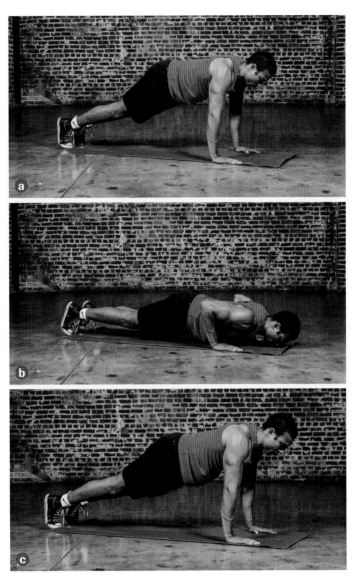

FIGURE 4.37 Press-up and hold.

REVERSE LUNGE WITH ROTATION

The reverse lunge with rotation tones the entire body with a focus on the legs and core. To begin, your feet should be shoulder-width apart and your torso up tall with arms at your sides and palms facing in (see figure 4.38a). Take a controlled lunge backwards with your left foot and raise your arms straight out in front of you (see figure 4.38b). Lower your hips so that your right thigh (front leg) becomes parallel to the floor. At this point your right knee should be directly over your ankle and your right foot should be pointing straight ahead, with your left knee bent at a 90-degree angle and pointing towards the floor. After reaching the bottom of the movement (when your left knee is 2.5 cm, or 1 in., from the floor), rotate your torso and arms over the leading leg (see figure 4.38c) and return to the centre. Return to the starting position and repeat on the other side.

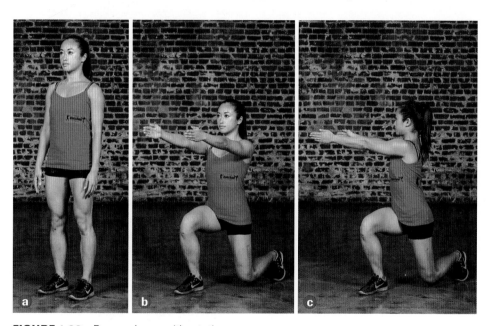

FIGURE 4.38 Reverse lunge with rotation.

SIDE-TO-SIDE LEAP

Standing with feet shoulder-width apart, load your body weight onto the left foot and raise the right foot off the floor (see figure 4.39a). Driving through the ball of the left foot, raise your arms overhead and leap as far as possible to the right (see figure 4.39b) so that you land on the right foot (see figure 4.39c). Returning to the starting position counts as one rep.

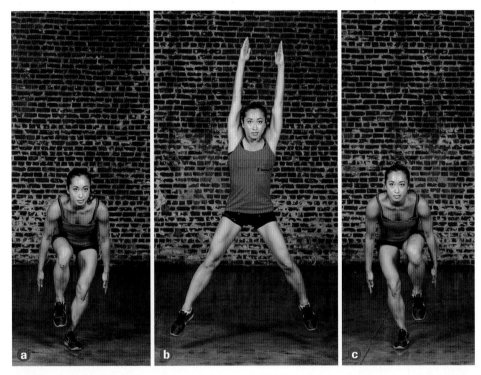

FIGURE 4.39 Side-to-side leap.

SINGLE-LEG WALL REACH

This exercise focuses on balance, coordination and flexibility. Stand on one foot about 5 to 7 centimetres (2 to 3 in.) from a wall. Rotate your body to reach with the opposite hand to three different areas on the wall (e.g., in front of you and to either side). You can increase the challenge by reaching high or low and mixing it up at random. Hold each position for 20 seconds (see figure 4.40, *a* through *d*). Throughout this exercise, maintain good posture and control your movement to maximise the benefits. Repeat on the other foot.

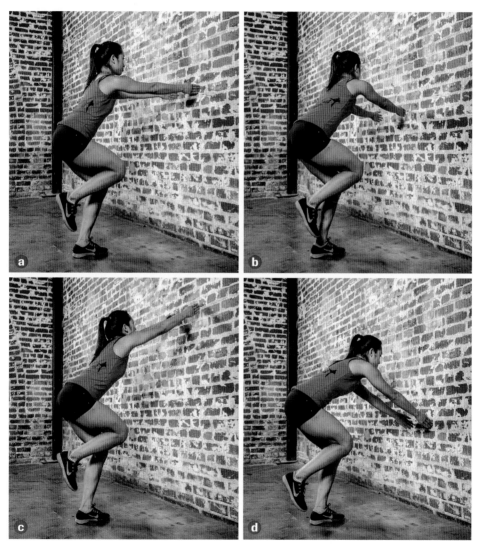

FIGURE 4.40 Single-leg wall reach: (*a*) front, (*b*) side, (*c*) high and (*d*) low.

SKIPPING

Skipping is a great tool to get your body warmed up for the main session of a Total Knockout Fitness workout. Here is a breakdown of the main skipping styles and techniques that will burn calories in no time and increase your cardiovascular fitness levels.

BACKWARD SKIPPING

Start the backward skipping technique by using your wrists to swing the rope over your head, but this time backwards, approaching your feet from behind you; take a small jump to allow the rope to pass beneath your feet. Then swing the rope up over your head again (backwards) and jump again when the rope approaches your feet from behind. Increase the speed of your jumps as you get more used to this exercise.

COMBINED HEEL-TOE TAP

Start the combined heel-toe tap by using your wrists to propel the rope over your head and towards your toes; take a small jump with the front of your right foot behind and the heel of your left foot in front to allow the rope to pass beneath your feet. Then swing the rope up over your head again and jump again when the rope approaches your toes, but this time tap the front of your left foot behind and the heel of your right foot in front. Increase the speed of your jumps as you get more used to this exercise.

CROSSOVER

Start the crossover technique by crossing your arms and using your wrists to swing the rope over your head and towards your toes; take a small jump to allow the rope to pass beneath your feet. Now uncross your arms, perform a normal single bounce skip and then cross your arms again. Then swing the rope up over your head again and jump again when the rope approaches your toes. Make sure your arms are crossed wide and low enough to step through the rope. Increase the speed of your jumps as you get more used to this exercise.

DOUBLE UNDER

Start the double under technique by using your wrists to swing the rope over your head and towards your toes; take two jumps (one jump over the rope followed by another jump when the rope is above your head). Increase the speed of your jumps as you get more used to this exercise.

HEEL TAP

Start the heel tap by using your wrists to swing the rope over your head and towards your toes; take a small jump with your feet together to allow the rope to pass beneath your feet. Then swing the rope up over your head again and jump again when the rope approaches your toes, but this time tap one heel in front. The third skip is performed with feet together; and the fourth skip, with one heel in front (alternate the feet you use to tap). Increase the speed of your jumps as you get more used to this exercise.

KNEE RAISE

Start the knee raise by using your wrists to swing the rope over your head and towards your toes; take a small jump with one knee raised to waist height to allow the rope to pass beneath your feet. Then swing the rope up over your head again and jump again, dropping your knee this time. Increase the speed of your jumps as you get more used to this exercise.

ONE TURN, TWO BOUNCES

Start the one turn, two bounces technique by using your wrists to swing the rope over your head and towards your toes; take two small, quick jumps to allow the rope to pass beneath your feet. Then swing the rope up over your head again and jump twice again when the rope approaches your toes.

SINGLE UNDER

Essentially, the single under technique is performed following this pattern: one turn of the rope for one bounce. Start this exercise by using your wrists to swing the rope over your head and towards your toes; take a small jump to allow the rope to pass beneath your feet. Then swing the rope up over your head again and jump again when it approaches your toes. Increase the speed of your jumps as you get more used to this exercise.

TOE TAP

Start the toe tap by using your wrists to swing the rope over your head and towards your toes; take a small jump with your feet together to allow the rope to pass beneath your feet. Then swing the rope up over your head again and jump again when the rope approaches your toes, but this time tap your toe behind. The third skip is performed with feet together; and the fourth skip, with toe behind (alternate the feet you use to tap). Increase the speed of your jumps as you get more used to this exercise.

TRIPLE UNDER

Start this exercise by using your wrists to swing the rope over your head and towards your toes; take three jumps and then allow the rope to pass beneath your feet. Then swing the rope up over your head again and continue this pattern. Increase the speed of your jumps as you get more used to this exercise.

SPIDERMAN CLIMB

This exercise increases flexibility in the glutes on the front-leg side and the hip flexors on the rear-leg side. Start in a press-up (also called a push-up) position (see figure 4.41a). Raise your left foot off the floor and bring the knee in towards the elbow (see figure 4.41b). Place your foot on the floor as close as possible to the outside of your hand (see figure 4.41c) Pause and hold this position for 20 to 30 seconds. Maintain good alignment with the rest of your body throughout this movement to ensure that your muscles are balanced. Then repeat on the other side.

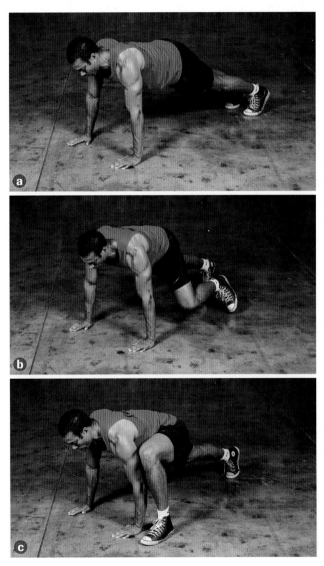

FIGURE 4.41 Spiderman climb.

SQUAT JUMP

The jumping squat is great for toning the core, bum, hips, thighs and calves. To perform the squat jump, start in an upright stance and midlevel guard (see round 6 for more details on how to perform a midlevel guard) with feet shoulder-width apart. Now step forwards with one foot, turn the rear foot 45 degrees, bend your knees, place your hand in the guard position and tuck your elbows in (see figure 4.42a). Inhale as you squat down by bending at the knees and sticking your butt back as you lower. Keep your head and chest up and your eyes looking forwards, and aim to get your thighs parallel to the floor. Exhale as you drive up through your heels and squeeze your butt (see figure 4.42b). As you leave the floor, rotate so you are in a mirrored stance as you land (see figure 4.42c) and repeat. If the squat jump is too difficult, you can perform squats without the jump.

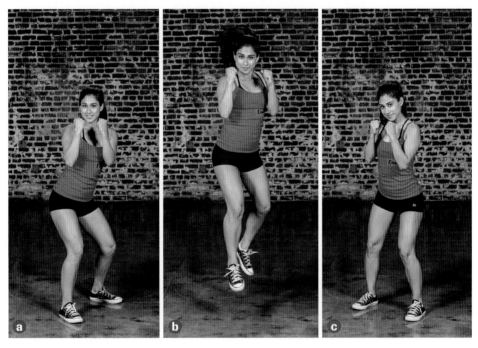

FIGURE 4.42 Squat jump.

TOE REACH AND TOUCH

This exercise improves balance and flexibility in the ankles, knees and hips. Stand on your right foot and, thinking of a clock face, reach out with your left foot to the 12 o'clock, 9 o'clock and, finally, 6 o'clock positions (see figure 4.43, *a* through *c*). Change feet and, with your right foot, reach out to the 12 o'clock, 3 o'clock and 6 o'clock positions. Repeat on each side.

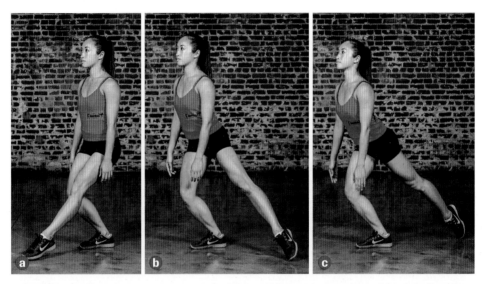

FIGURE 4.43   Toe reach and touch with the left foot: (*a*) 12 o'clock position, (*b*) 9 o'clock position and (*c*) 6 o'clock position.

TOTAL-BODY TRAINING STRETCH

Remember to complete your workout with a two-minute total-body training stretch to allow your body to recover from the main session. The total-body training stretch includes the hamstring and calf stretch for 20 to 30 seconds with each leg, the outward and inward shoulder stretch for 20 to 30 seconds for each shoulder and the lying knee to chest for 20 seconds with each leg.

TOY SOLDIER MARCH

The toy soldier march activates the hamstrings, glutes and hip flexors. Start in a standing position (see figure 4.44a); keeping your left leg straight, kick it up in front of you as high as you can (see figure 4.44b). Touch your toes with the fingertips of your right arm; this is basically a straight-leg march. Repeat with the right leg.

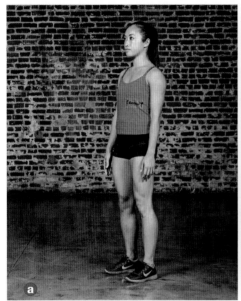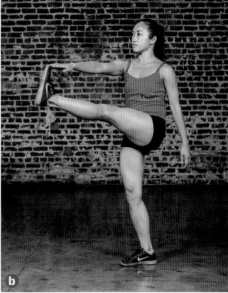

FIGURE 4.44 Toy soldier march.

TRICEPS DIP

The triceps dip is great for toning the backs of your arms. Position yourself in front of a bench, or step, with your hands shoulder-width apart, your knees bent and your feet about hip-width apart on the floor in front of you. Straighten your arms to support your body weight and keep a little bend in your elbows to maintain the tension in your triceps and protect your elbow joints (see figure 4.45a). Now slowly bend at your elbows and lower your body towards the floor until your arms are at about a 90-degree angle (see figure 4.45b). Be sure to keep your back and bum close to the bench. Return to the starting position under control and repeat.

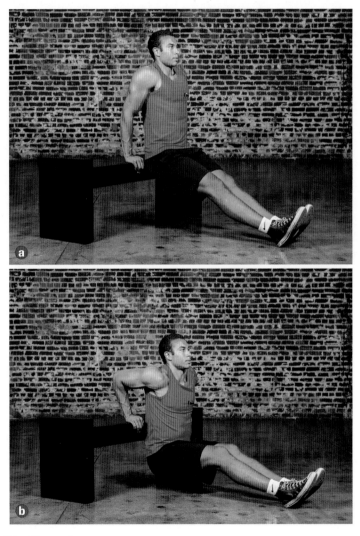

FIGURE 4.45 Triceps dip.

TUCK JUMP

Stand with your feet shoulder-width apart (see figure 4.46a). Jump up as high as you can, throwing your arms up; while in the air, quickly tuck your legs in towards your chest before landing (see figure 4.46b). Quickly extend your legs to absorb the landing. Keep your chest up and maintain good posture throughout.

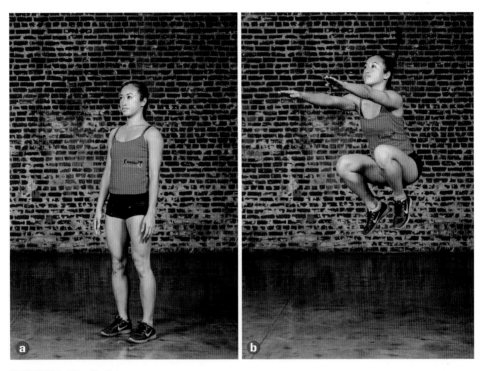

FIGURE 4.46   Tuck jump.

WALKING LUNGE

This movement works your glutes, hamstrings and quadriceps as well as your abdominal, back and core muscles as you work to keep your balance. The walking lunge is the same as a normal lunge, except that you propel yourself forwards with each lunge. Stand facing forwards with your feet shoulder-width apart (see figure 4.47a). Keep your back straight and your head and chin up. You can place your hands on your hips while you do your walking lunges. Lift your right foot up in a 90-degree angle, and have your leg form an upside-down L. Keep your knee and hip aligned, as well as your knee and ankle. Inhale as you step forwards with your heel landing first. Roll your foot down until your toes touch the floor. Lower your back knee so that it almost touches the floor (see figure 4.47b). When in the lunge position, keep your knee and hips aligned and your knee and ankle aligned, and don't allow your front knee to extend beyond your toes. Exhale as you use your weight and push up off your back toes. Push your body forwards to land your back foot in front to do another lunge, moving forwards with each lunge. Pushing up off your back leg and moving it forwards to the next lunge should occur in one continuous motion.

To perform an advanced walking lunge, hold a weight (ideally between 2 and 4 kg, or 4.4 and 8.8 lb) in each hand or use a barbell to increase the challenge. This will improve your strength by increasing the intensity of your warm-up. Once your technique is correct and you feel less challenged by the weight in your hands, you can increase it. Adding weight is not the most important part of this exercise, however; the technique is most crucial. Stabilise yourself with your heel and push down, making sure that your back foot meets the floor or ground.

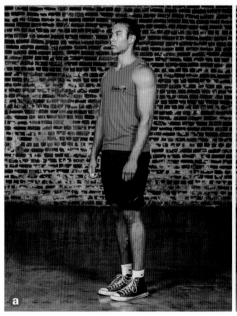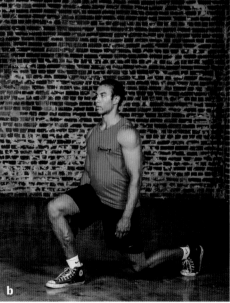

FIGURE 4.47 Walking lunge.

WALKING QUAD STRETCH

The walking quad stretch is ideal for loosening and stretching the quadriceps and hip flexors. Start from a standing position (see figure 4.48*a*). Hold the right ankle with the right hand and pull the heel to the glute with the knee pointed to the ground for around 30 seconds as the left hip and ankle extend (see figure 4.48*b*). Keep the glute contracted during the stretch, and do not hyperextend the lower back. Breathe deeply to allow the muscles to stretch deeply. Step forwards with right foot and repeat the stretch on the other side. Continue, alternating legs.

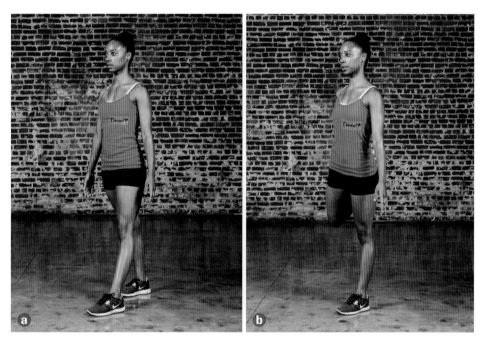

FIGURE 4.48 Walking quad stretch.

ROUND 5

Warm-Ups

Warming up to prepare your body for a workout is vital to avoid injury and can reduce the amount of muscle soreness in the days following your workout. There are many ways to get your body warmed up for boxing, and some are definitely more effective than others. The Total Knockout Fitness warm-up, created by top boxing champions and fitness experts, combines dynamic stretching with fun skipping techniques (plus a few other techniques) so you can make the most of your exercise routine and have the energy you need for everyday life. It was especially designed to get you ready for a calorie-busting, toning workout that raises your energy and fitness levels and conveys the following benefits:

✔ Allows your muscles to relax and contract faster during your main workout because they are warmed up and focused on working harder, which will help you shape and tone your body in just the right places.

✔ Improves your overall performance and experience of your workout by preparing your whole body for the main session.

✔ Loosens up your muscles to reduce the risk of injury and muscle soreness by gradually preparing your body for the more vigorous activity that follows.

✔ Enhances range of motion, strength and speed by stimulating your muscles' motor units.

✔ Raises your body temperature, which improves the elasticity of your muscles and reduces the risk of getting pulls and strains.

✔ Increases your heart rate slowly to get your heart ready for exercise.

✔ Increases your mental focus by clearing your mind. This focuses your mind and body on exercise and using your muscles in all the right ways.

The Total Knockout Fitness programmes outlined later in this book are typically 60 minutes long and divided into three parts: the warm-up (which usually lasts around 10 minutes), the main session (lasting around 45 minutes) and the cool-down (lasting approximately 5 minutes). This setup ensures that the body is ready for what is to come at all times. During the warm-up the body is prepared for the demands of the main session of the workout. The main session gives way to the relaxation and calming of the muscles and body in the cool-down phase to bring about the full benefits of the workout and reduce the risk of muscle soreness the next day.

This round explores fun and simple tools to help you fully enjoy and benefit from a champion warm-up that gets your body and mind prepared for calorie-busting boxing moves and styles that will get you sweating in no time and burn calories at high speed. Three standard 10-minute warm-up routines are included: basic, advanced and ultimate. Once you are confident and have mastered all of the stretches and skipping skills, feel free to experiment with and mix the techniques to create a warm-up that suits your needs and preferences and challenges you. Changing your warm-up routines to ones with greater challenge will keep them fun, fresh and exciting.

Preparing for the Total Knockout Fitness Workout

Before you start with your Total Knockout Fitness warm-up, make sure you are ready for it—with mind and body. This will help you make the most of it and feel the benefits of your exercise routine right from the start. Have a look at the following tips for getting ready for your warm-up.

Drink and Eat Two Hours Before Your Workout

Make sure you are hydrated and topped up with a light and nutritious meal *at least two hours* before you start your workout. Eating too close to the time you start working out may leave you lethargic and unable to respond to the exercise at the optimum level. Opt for foods that give you a balanced combination of protein and carbohydrate and are easy to digest. For example, you could enjoy an avocado or tuna spread on a slice of wholemeal bread, or banana and almonds mixed with yoghurt. If you fancy a slightly bigger snack, opt for chicken breast with couscous. Don't forget to take in enough fluid: about one or two glasses of water or an isotonic drink. Avoid fruits that are acidic such as kiwis and oranges because they may leave your stomach feeling uncomfortable when working out. In addition, stay away from fatty foods such as pizza, burgers, deep-fried foods and sweets, and reduce or avoid starchy foods such as bread, pasta, potatoes and rice. Working out on a heavy stomach can make you feel sick and inflexible.

Set the Scene

Prepare everything you need for your workout before you start your warm-up. You don't want to have to interrupt your warm-up or main session to get a drink, switch on the radio, get a towel or change your clothes.

If you work out at home, make sure you have the room you plan to do your workout in all set up and that you won't be interrupted by roommates, partners or children. To remain focused during a warm-up and main session, you may prefer an atmosphere that is free of disturbances. A quiet spot in the boxing area of a gym buzzing with activity or an allocated studio space may work.

If music motivates you when working out, load up your favourite tracks, take out all the exercise equipment you need (e.g., skipping ropes, boxing gloves), change into some loose-fitting exercise clothes (a simple T-shirt and shorts will do just fine, nothing fancy is required here), take out a hand towel for those sweaty moments you should experience in every session and don't forget to bring along this book to guide you through your workout until the routine is completely rehearsed. After a while you won't require the guidelines because the routines will become second nature; you will also discover the programmes and routines that work best for you and begin to do them automatically. If at some stage you are looking for new inspiration and a change in your exercise routine, simply pick up this guide again for fresh ideas to work your body into shape.

Warm Up Your Mind

You can use your warm-up to get your body and mind completely focused on what is still to come: a calorie-busting exercise routine that will help you achieve your fitness and body goals—closer and closer with every move you make. Total Knockout Fitness's elite performance coaches who train high-level athletes know that mental preparation is vital to a balanced and optimal workout.

Get Super-Motivated Before You Start

Think about the motivations behind your workouts before you even start warming up. Ask yourself why you are about to have a workout, and think about the changes it will bring about. Do you want to lose weight to look and feel slimmer? Do you aspire to a more toned, stronger body? Remind yourself of your goals before you commence your warm-up, and remember that every repetition is getting you closer to that goal! This will keep you focused on your desired outcomes and get your mind in the right place from the start.

Total Knockout Fitness Warm-Up Techniques

The warm-ups you are about to enjoy have been specifically designed by leading celebrity trainers and boxing champions to provide an all-around routine that will prepare your body for the Total Knockout Fitness main session. They include fun moves and exercises that will get your heart rate up and warm your muscles so you get the most out of your workout. Following is more detail about these techniques.

Skipping

Don't we all love the one thing boxing gyms all over the world have in common: the whistling sounds of rapidly spinning ropes. For most boxers and fitness lovers, that's the sound of a good, genuine workout that provides great results. A highly effective way to boost fitness, skipping has the following benefits:

✔ It is a great muscle toner, shaping your legs and increasing their power, which you need to perform good footwork.

✔ It increases mobility, eye–hand coordination, reflexes and balance.

✔ It develops endurance and stamina.

✔ It improves rhythm, agility and footwork.

The Total Knockout Fitness training programmes integrate about five minutes of fun skipping techniques into the warm-up. Skipping prepares your body in all the right areas for a workout that includes vigorous boxing activity. It strengthens the muscles in your legs, improves your posture and raises your heart rate and is a great cardiorespiratory tool. Before you get started, have a quick look at the types of skipping ropes available.

Here are some extra tips to get your skipping technique right—from the start! Before you start skipping, bear in mind the following:

✔ Your back should be straight and your shoulders square; your legs should be slightly bent at the knees to avoid injury.

✔ Don't jump too high! A soft jump will do the job just fine and ensure that you land safely back on the ground.

Skipping to your favourite tunes will make your training a lot more fun. Without realising it, you could even find yourself working harder (scientists have proven that music positively influences exercise). Music may also improve your timing and coordination, so turn on your iPod, MP3 player or sound system and start skipping away to your classics.

✔ Always start at a slow pace and work your way up gradually.

✔ Whatever type of skipping rope you choose, remember to buy the right size. Table 1.1 in round 1 can help you with this.

✔ Skip on a rubberised gym floor, wooden floor or carpeted floor wearing running, cross-training or boxing shoes.

✔ Skip in front of a full-length mirror, especially at the beginning of your skipping experience, so you can see your movements.

✔ Avoid looking down at your feet as this can disturb your timing.

✔ Keep your elbows tucked in to your sides.

✔ Use your wrists to make sure the rope turns smoothly

✔ Don't lean forwards; keep your head up and your back straight.

✔ Try not to skip too slowly to keep your feet from catching on the rope.

✔ When skipping, keep the rope tight at all times.

✔ If you are speed jumping, use small jumps, keeping the rope close to your head.

Dynamic Stretching

At Total Knockout Fitness we integrate dynamic stretches and advanced dynamic stretches into every warm-up to maximise the fitness benefits of boxing. Unlike static stretching, which is performed while standing still, dynamic stretching is performed while moving. Because it increases range of movement and blood and oxygen flow to soft tissues, dynamic stretching prepares the body for physical exertion and sport performance. Dynamic stretching is now used by most coaches and sport professionals to improve performance and reduce the risk of injury. It both prepares the body for an effective workout and helps muscles to relax after an exercise routine.

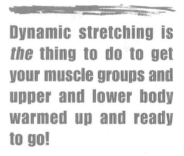

Dynamic stretching is *the* thing to do to get your muscle groups and upper and lower body warmed up and ready to go!

Total Knockout Fitness Warm-Up Routines

Here they are—figures 5.1, 5.2 and 5.3 provide the Total Knockout Fitness warm-up routines that will get you super-ready for the main session. Note that you will find all of the exercises listed in these workouts in round 4.

Start with the easiest, basic routine and advance as you become more confident with the more complicated skipping and dynamic stretching routines. When starting out, stick to 10 reps of each warm-up exercise to

FIGURE 5.1 Basic Warm-Up

Skipping	Single under (10 reps) Double under (10 reps)
Dynamic stretching	Lunge (30 seconds) High-knees running (30 seconds) Toy soldier march (30 seconds)
Other techniques	Jog on the spot (30 sec) Press-up (10 reps)
Total time: approximately 10 min	

FIGURE 5.2 Intermediate Warm-Up

Skipping	Single under (10 reps) Double under (10 reps) Backward skipping (10 reps)
Dynamic stretching	Advanced walking lunge (10 reps) Toy soldier march (30 sec) Over the fence (30 sec)
Other techniques	Jog on the spot (30 sec) Press-up (10 reps)
Total time: approximately 10 min	

FIGURE 5.3 Advanced Warm-Up

Skipping	Backward skipping (10 reps) Crossover (10 reps) Heel tap (10 reps)
Dynamic stretching	Advanced walking lunge (10 reps) Glute kick (10 reps) Over the fence (10 reps)
Other techniques	Jog on the spot (30 sec) Press-up (10 reps)
Total time: approximately 10 min	

get your body used to its new level of activity slowly and step by step. As your fitness level increases and you feel you want to push your body a bit harder, attempt 15 reps of each exercise. Because you will be faster at doing the exercises and stretches, your warm-up won't be any longer. You just do a lot more in less time, which is a brilliant thing if you want to burn more calories!

Take time to learn and master all of the basic warm-up techniques before moving on to more advanced routines.

Well done. You have completed the first set of physical exercises in this book. You now have a pretty good idea of how to get your body ready for the main workout session that is still to come. Regardless of how excited you get about throwing punches in style and speed in the coming rounds, always ensure that you start your exercise sessions with a good, balanced warm-up. It will help your body fully benefit from the boxing moves you will learn in the following rounds.

ROUND 6

Form and Footwork

You now know about the equipment you can use to make the most of boxing for fitness, and you have learned how healthy nutrition can optimise your boxing workout routines and how balanced warm-up techniques can enhance your main workout session. Now it is time to get down to it and start with the practical, fun part of using boxing techniques to get you in tiptop shape and bring your knockout physique to light!

This round explores the foundations of boxing, including the movements everyone—from novice to champion—needs to get right: the stance, guard (arm position) and footwork. You will learn boxing techniques that will boost your fitness level and tone your body—moves and footwork skills that will set you up for calorie-burning, head-turning footwork and punch combinations.

Getting the fundamentals of boxing right is beyond important. You can't run before you learn to walk, and the same is true in boxing. You must learn and master the basic boxing movements before progressing to the execution of punches and combinations. Here are a few key reasons for getting the basics right.

Get the Basics Right From the Start

Boxing basics, from the correct stance and guard position to basic footwork, provide a sound, safe foundation to work from so you can excel in more advanced boxing skills and drills. They equip you with the core knowledge of how to position and move your body to execute boxing skills safely and confidently. Mastering these basics also prepares you for the techniques and demands of the four key punches you will learn about in round 7 by making sure your hands and feet, back and legs are positioned optimally to perform good punches.

Getting the basics right also protects you from injury to the shoulders, lower spine and joints when throwing punches and carrying out other boxing moves. A safe and correct stance prevents injury to the wrists, elbows and shoulders and lower spine and enables you to throw punch combinations efficiently and accurately time after time. Good and safe footwork allows you to move smoothly and swiftly in all directions while also increasing your punch power and speed. When you have 70 percent of your weight on the balls of your feet and are leaning slightly forwards from the hips, your body weight transfers forwards giving you extra power to punch. This allows you to rely less on strength and more on body weight and movement.

Boost Your Cardiorespiratory Fitness Level

Acquiring correct boxing fundamentals also boosts your cardiorespiratory fitness level. Fast and safe footwork and the ability to make quick switches from various stance and guard positions will get your heart rate up and burn calories, helping to burn fat and increase muscle endurance, which in turn will create a leaner physique. Positioning yourself safely and most effectively will give you a solid foundation from which to consistently improve the quality of your movements and, eventually, your punches. As your fitness level improves over the coming weeks, you will naturally be able to throw more punches, your movements will become quicker and easier and you will burn more calories.

Get Toned

Form and footwork exercises will not only help you execute dynamic punch combos swiftly and smoothly, but also tone and shape your legs and accelerate your metabolism. You will burn more calories while developing core muscles in your abdomen, lower back, upper arms and shoulders.

Now that you know all the benefits of creating a strong foundation of basic boxing skills, let's get started on learning how to go about it. This round addresses all you need to know about the basic stance, guard and footwork techniques. Make sure you follow the techniques step by step and practise them over and over until you get them right 100 percent of the time and could do them in your sleep.

Stance

Usually, the first technique new boxers learn is the stance because it is the foundation from which they will perform all of the other boxing moves. We use a specific training system called 'from the ground up', which means that the ground is your leverage point for all the movements you are going to perform. Having a strong, stable base and a balanced body allows you to move in all directions with ease, balance, speed, power and precision. If your stance is not correct, you will have difficulty performing punches and footwork safely and effectively. Practising the stance correctly from the beginning, and over and over, is crucial for getting the most out of your exercise routines and achieving your fitness, weight and energy goals.

First of all, you should establish whether you are more naturally an orthodox (right-handed, therefore leading with the left foot) or southpaw (left-handed, therefore leading with the right foot). To assume the proper stance, begin with a step forwards at walking pace with your lead foot, keeping your feet in line with your shoulders and shift your body weight forward so that 70 percent of your weight is on the balls of your feet. Turn the back foot out 45 degrees and lean slightly forwards from the hips. Shifting your body weight to the balls of your feet as you throw punches helps you maintain soft knees, or knees that are slightly bent. Note that if you are right-handed, your left shoulder should be pointed towards the target; if you are left-handed, your right shoulder should be pointed towards the target. When executing a stance, remind yourself that your back should remain fairly straight. If you're struggling, try assuming the stance in front of a mirror.

Three stance positions are commonly used in boxing: upright, semi-crouch and full crouch. Professional boxers are encouraged to use all of them at different times and change them throughout their performance to keep their opponents guessing. In this programme, however, we use only the upright stance because it is most beneficial in terms of fitness and posture.

To execute the upright stance, as shown in figure 6.1, stand with your legs shoulder-width apart and make sure your lead foot is a half step in front of the rear foot (note that right-handed, also called orthodox, boxers lead with the left foot and fist). The right hand is at chin level and the lead (left) fist is held vertically about 15 centimetres (6 in.) in front of the face at chin level. The rear (right) fist is held beside the chin and the elbow is positioned 8 to 10 centimetres (3 to 4 in.) from the rib cage in a naturally relaxed position to protect the body. The chin is slightly tucked into the chest without touching it and held slightly off-centre. This is to avoid punches to the jaw that commonly cause knockouts in the sport of boxing.

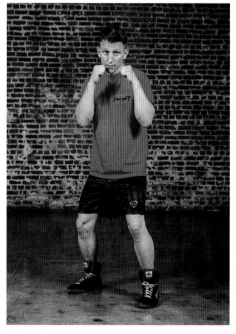

FIGURE 6.1 Upright stance.

Guard

The guard (i.e., the positioning of the arms and hands in proportion the head) ensures the protection of the chin, face and upper body; rotating the shoulders to move the arms up and down provides this protection. The benefits of maintaining a good guard in Total Knockout Fitness are strengthened muscles around the shoulders; this, combined with the increased strength that results from the other movements and exercises, can considerably improve your posture.

Three of the guard styles used in boxing are the high, or peek-a-boo, guard; the low guard; and the midlevel guard. The midlevel guard, in which the fists are in line with the jaw, allows you to move your hands up as high as your temple and to move your elbows down to cover the complete rib cage. This is the primary guard style you will use in the Total Knockout Fitness programme, and it will keep your head and face protected throughout the boxing training.

> Go back to the basics and practise the guard and stance as often as possible. As the programme progresses, you'll realise just how important it is to get these basics right. It will help you hugely when learning the punches.

Start the guard in a good upright stance position as explained at the beginning of this round. To cover, or protect, your ribs, bring your elbows close to your sides and raise your forearms at the same time. Bring your fists in line with your chin. Relax your arms and keep your body relaxed until the point of impact. Lean your head slightly forwards, keep your hands at chin level and turn your palms inwards. This creates a perfect stance and guard. Distribute your weight equally between both feet. Do not tip forwards onto the balls of your feet. Always keep your shoulders and arms relaxed when in guard position. After throwing a punch, always bring your arms and hands back into guard position. See figure 6.2 for an example of the midlevel guard.

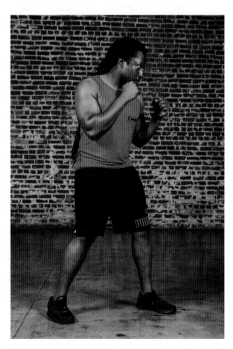

FIGURE 6.2   Midlevel guard.

Footwork

Now that you have the tools and know-how to maintain a good guard and stance, we turn to the skill that the world-famous boxer, Muhammad Ali, was known for: footwork! Footwork refers to the specific movement of the feet; good footwork allows you to move in all directions quickly and smoothly and is the foundation for throwing accurate punches. With good footwork you will burn more calories and be able to change direction very quickly. It improves your balance, giving you a lot more speed, power and accuracy with both single punches and combinations. Balance is critical in boxing, and an integral part of balance is footwork. Bad footwork will put you off balance resulting in weaker punches.

Keeping Your Balance

In boxing, the better you are at staying balanced, the more confident you will be and the stronger and more accurate your punches will be. So the question is, how can you practise maintaining and improving your balance?

> Keep the gap between your legs at shoulder width or slightly wider; a narrow gap could cause you to lose balance. Widen the gap as you move forwards or backwards, and then return to stance position. At no time should you cross your feet or keep them parallel to each other.

> Place 70 percent of your weight on the balls of your feet.

> Contact the floor lightly.

> Balance your body weight equally through both legs until the point of impact.

> Take small steps when focusing on footwork.

> Check your feet! When your feet are not in the proper position, you can lose balance, lack power and compromise your defense.

> Assume a proper stance. Keep the feet roughly shoulder-width apart and the knees slightly bent. To test the balance of a stance, have someone push you relatively hard. If you lose your balance, your stance is not solid.

> When performing footwork drills, do not move your feet without moving your head and arms accordingly. Your body should move fluidly back and forth in a solid stance.

> Don't overpunch. Putting too much force behind a punch can throw you off balance. Throw punches with controlled power while maintaining a stable stance.

> Use shadowboxing to improve footwork and balance. Shadowboxing is boxing against air and is an excellent way to improve your balance.

> Improve your fitness. If you lack fitness and conditioning, your mobility, footwork and balance will be the first things to suffer.

This section explains how to integrate footwork skills into your stance and guard to improve your technique as well as your speed, agility and flexibility. In addition, one of the main outcomes of good footwork skills is being in the flow of punching on the move, which maximises your reactivity, speed and flow of movement (we'll discuss this in more detail later in this round and in round 7). Good footwork is also critical in power generation because you can punch without losing your balance.

Once you understand these key things about balanced footwork, you have the basics to avoid injury and begin to move with speed and precision. The next section addresses moving in specific directions to burn calories and solidify the boxing basics.

Moving Forwards and Backwards

When throwing punches, moving forwards gives you more impact because your body weight adds to the power of the punch. If an opponent is advancing you, you may want to move backwards and throw punches while doing so. The force that propels the movement always starts form the opposite foot to the direction in which you are about to move. When you are moving forwards, the push comes from the back foot. The front foot moves first (see figure 6.3a) and the back foot follows an equal distance (see figure 6.3b). When moving backwards, the push comes from the front foot. The back foot moves first (see figure 6.4a) and the front foot follows an equal distance (see figure 6.4b). Just remember, whether you are moving forwards or backwards, to keep your steps at a normal walking pace. Practise moving forwards and then backwards until you feel confident in the movement. It may take a while.

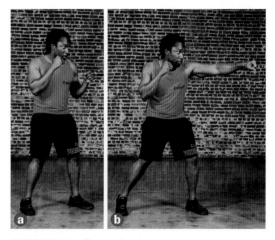
FIGURE 6.3 Forward movement.

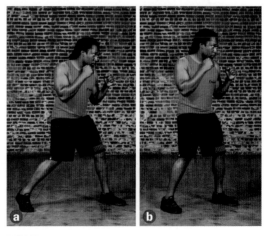
FIGURE 6.4 Backward movement.

Moving Side-to-Side

In boxing for fitness, lateral (side-to-side) movement is good for activating the adductor and abductor muscles as you are pushing off the balls of your feet. In professional boxing you can throw a wider variety of punches and punch combinations with a higher potential of penetrating your opponent's guard. The side-to-side movement is also used when counterpunching or trying to avoid incoming shots from an opponent. Generally, orthodox (right-handed) boxers prefer to move to the left side because it is the most natural movement as they push off the right leg and slide to the left. This is because the left foot is much closer to the opponent. Left-handed boxers usually prefer to move to the right side. Always remember that the push comes from the opposite foot to the direction in which you are about to move. If you are moving left, the push comes form the right foot. The left foot moves first and the right foot follows an equal distance. If you are moving right, the push comes from the left foot. The right foot moves first and the left foot follows an equal distance (see figure 6.5 for a view of the side-to-side movement going left). The back foot functions as the power driver, allowing you to push forwards in fast attack. Note that your front foot always needs to remain towards your opponent. At the same time it needs to be in line with the target. Practise this until it is second nature. It will keep you one step ahead in your Total Knockout Fitness programme.

> To get your footwork right from the start, make sure you have mastered the stance and guard, which will support you in learning to move forwards and backwards and to the left and right smoothly to ensure quick, smooth, flowing movements!

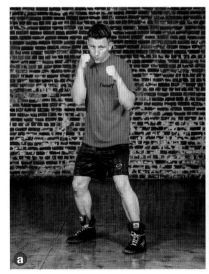
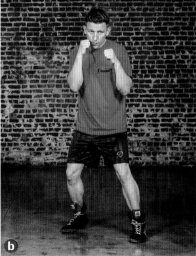

FIGURE 6.5 Side-to-side movement going left.

Shuffling

Boxers shuffle to encourage their opponents to 'chase' them so they will tire. Shuffling involves rocking the body from side to side, slightly bending the knees and pushing off the back foot to slide forwards. See figure 6.6 for an example of shuffling.

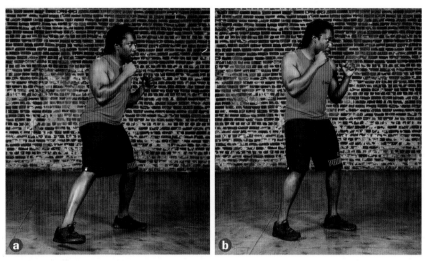

FIGURE 6.6 Shuffling movement.

Changing Direction

When you can change direction in boxing, you will have more options for attacking, counterpunching and defending, thereby throwing opponents off balance or catching them off guard. Changing direction requires a move called pivoting. Start by shifting your body weight onto the ball of the foot of the leading leg; use the back leg to push you in a circular motion, and then turn the rest of your body to the new target. A usual range is 15 to 45 degrees. See figure 6.7 for an example of the pivot movement used to change direction.

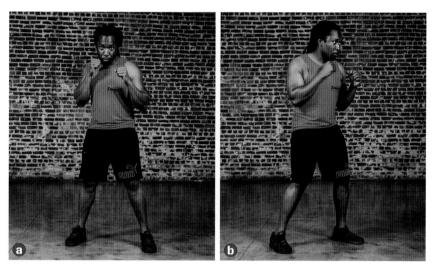

FIGURE 6.7 Pivot movement used to change direction.

2-2-2-2 Pattern

To add some fun and burn calories at high speed, you will learn some simple Total Knockout Fitness movement patterns. These will improve your coordination and balance and get your whole body moving with energy.

When shuffling, you can follow the same technique as those used when moving forwards and backwards and laterally. These techniques accustom you to basic footwork and bring awareness to your balance. Before making a shuffle, move your body naturally backwards and forwards using small movements. Then move your legs backwards and forwards with slightly bent knees and push off the balls of your feet, take half a step and then, in quick succession, another half step. Getting used to moving your body weight around will improve the power and accuracy of your punches.

The 2-2-2-2 pattern exercise is as follows:

> Move forwards two shuffles.

> Move backwards two shuffles.

> Move two shuffles to the left.

> Move two shuffles to the right.

Begin this movement slowly, and make sure you maintain the triangular Total Knockout Fitness base. Keep your feet as close to the floor as possible throughout, always making sure that the main movement of your legs is a shuffle, not a jump. Do this for 40 to 60 seconds, repeating three times while remembering to focus on the correct movement and maintain your base so you are using your body efficiently.

Form and Footwork Drills and Exercises

This section outlines some exercises and drills you can use to master your form and footwork and improve your speed, power and agility.

COMBINATION DRILL

The combination drill is a great way to combine footwork, stance and guard in one fluid movement, while getting your heart rate up and starting to burn calories and fat—for a healthier, more energetic body. Start in the upright stance and guard positions. Now move backwards and forwards, remembering that you push off the back foot and slide the front foot to go forwards and push off the front foot and slide the back foot to go backwards. Repeat this for three minutes; then take a break and repeat for another three minutes. If you have the hang of it already, congratulations! If you need a bit more practice, simply go a few more rounds until you feel confident in your movement and can perform all three techniques in one swift, smooth movement.

You can practise this exercise as part of your main session whenever you need a reminder of how to put the boxing basics together and perform integrated footwork in the stance and guard position. Not only will it improve your footwork, but it will also tone your legs and glutes; it's definitely worth the pearls of sweat!

FAST FOOTWORK DRILL

The fast footwork drill focuses on getting your footwork faster and more precise, enabling you to improve your side-to-side movement skills as well as strengthening the muscles in your lower body. In an upright stance with your feet shoulder-width apart, step at a walking pace forward with your lead foot, keeping your feet in line with your shoulders and rotating your back foot 45 degrees (see figure 6.8*a*). Move forward by pushing off with the rear foot (see figure 6.8*b*), move to the right by pushing off with the left foot (see figure 6.8*c*), and then try to move back to the left by pushing off with the right foot (see figure 6.8*d*). Now throw your weight from the left to the right foot. Repeat 5 to 10 times. Once you have confidence in the movement, repeat with exaggerated movements.

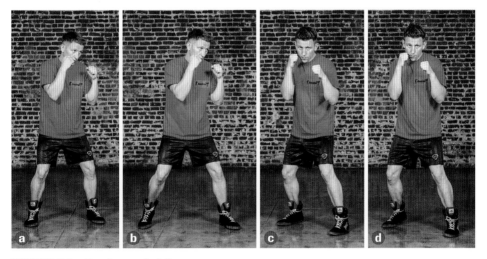

FIGURE 6.8   Fast footwork drill.

ON THE MOVE DRILL

The on the move drill allows you to throw punches while on the move and burn calories while strengthening the muscles in the upper and lower body. As in the previous drill, start in an upright stance with your feet shoulder-width apart and step at a walking pace, keeping your feet in line with your shoulders and rotating the back foot 45 degrees. Move forward by pushing off with the rear foot, move to the right by pushing off with the left foot, and then try to move back to the left by pushing off with the right foot. Initially you should concentrate on just the footwork for this drill, but after you learn punches in the next round, you can change up the drill by executing punches as you move. Repeat 10 times, rest for 5 seconds and repeat 15 times.

PARTNER FOOTWORK DRILL

Training with a partner can be hugely beneficial in getting your boxing basics on point. It can give you that extra boost of motivation to get the most out of the workout and push you a bit harder to burn more calories and ultimately have a better experience. When training with a partner, try these moves:

> Move forwards and backwards, left and right, while your partner tries to mirror your movements.
> Move in a circular motion around your partner.
> Shift and shuffle your feet quickly, mirroring your partner.

SHUFFLE FOOTWORK DRILL

For the shuffle footwork drill, bring your attention to your foot position and maintain good balance through your triangular base with 70 percent of your body weight on the balls of your feet. Perform two 2-minute rounds of the following with 45-second rests between rounds (when proficient, increase to three shuffles):

> Two shuffles forwards
> Two shuffles backwards
> Two shuffles left
> Two shuffles right

SHUFFLE-DUCK FOOTWORK DRILL

The following exercise allows for a progression of the preceding by adding a defensive move called the duck. This requires greater effort from the lower-body muscle groups (i.e., legs and butt), ultimately toning these areas of your body. To perform a duck, begin in an upright stance and sit your body weight down into your legs and butt lowering your shoulder height by 12-14 inches. Then, drive up through the floor to return to the initial upright stance. For the shuffle-duck footwork drill, perform the following pattern:

> Two forward shuffles-duck-two backwards shuffles-duck
> Two left shuffles-duck-two right shuffles-duck

Or, as an alternative, perform the following pattern:

> Three forward shuffles-three backward shuffles-three left shuffles-three right shuffles
> Two forward shuffles-duck-two backward shuffles-duck
> Two left shuffles-duck-two right shuffles-duck

LADDER DRILL

Using ladders improves your agility and your ability to change directions quickly. Another way to get your feet working is speed ladders, a technique used in many evasion, power/speed or team sports. These are laid on the ground and you step into each rung of the ladder sharply, raising your knees on each step (see figure 6.9, *a* and *b*). This trains the leg muscles and improves cardiorespiratory fitness.

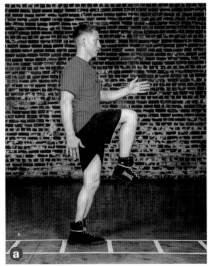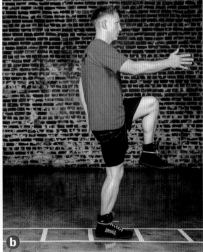

FIGURE 6.9 Ladder drill.

FOOTWORK CLOCK DRILL

The footwork clock drill includes two change-of-direction exercises that keep you working on your feet constantly and also help you improve your concentration. A more focused mind produces better results for your body and ultimately your fitness level—the number one thing we focus on in this programme. Once your mind is completely focused and you are concentrating fully on the exercises, you will realize your body will perform them with ease and speed, allowing you to burn more calories.

For the first exercise, start in the middle of an imaginary circle of about 10 metres in diameter or clock face where 12 o'clock is ahead of you. A partner shouts a number from 1 to 12, and you sprint to that hour of the clock and then back to the middle. Keep focused on the hours of the clock and the directions you need to head in. Because your training partner is shouting a number as soon as you get back to the centre of the clock, you have no idea where you will be heading next.

As in the first exercise, in this one, you are standing at the centre of an imaginary clock face. This time, however, you are in boxing stance (with your guard up as normal) and the circle is much smaller, about 5 metres in diameter. When your training partner calls out a number, you take one shuffle (maintaining your boxing stance at all times) in that direction before returning to the middle and then heading in the direction of the next number called. If you are doing this exercise correctly, you will be working nonstop for the entire round—constantly on your toes and always moving. Start with four 1-minute rounds to create a solid base, but work up to four to six 2-minute rounds.

Total Knockout Fitness Ultimate Form and Footwork Workouts

There are three levels of form and footwork workouts that are provided: a basic form and footwork workout, an intermediate form and footwork workout and an advanced form and footwork workout.

Basic Ultimate Form and Footwork Workout

The basic form and footwork workout in figure 6.10 provides a solid foundation on how to get the stance, guard and footwork right from the start. This workout focuses on increasing your sense of balance as well as providing you with techniques to burn calories with fun footwork drills that will also strengthen your legs and improve your posture. When you are able to perform the basic workout with ease it is time to move on to the intermediate workout.

FIGURE 6.10   **Basic Ultimate Form and Footwork Workout**

Warm-up	Perform the basic warm-up, intermediate warm-up or advanced warm-up from round 5.
Movements	Practise the forward and backward movement for 1 min followed by 1 min of shuffling movements.
Combination drill	Perform for 3 min; then take a break and repeat for another 3 min.
Fast footwork drill	Repeat 5 times.
On the move drill	Perform 10 times, rest for 5 seconds and repeat 15 times.
Ladder drill	Perform for 2 min.
Cool-down	Hamstring and calf stretch (20-30 sec each leg); outward and inward shoulder stretch (20-30 sec each shoulder); and lying knee to chest (20 sec each leg)

Intermediate Ultimate Form and Footwork Workout

The intermediate form and footwork workout in figure 6.11 will challenge your body even further with slightly longer exercise duration, allowing your body to work harder and longer to get the benefits of improved posture, more confidence in executing the stance, guard and footwork skills, while burning more calories for enhanced weight loss and increased cardio fitness.

FIGURE 6.11   **Intermediate Ultimate Form and Footwork Workout**

Warm-up	Perform the basic warm-up, intermediate warm-up or advanced warm-up from round 5.
Movements	Practise the forward and backward movement for 1 min followed by 1.5 min of shuffling movements.
Combination drill	Perform for 3 min; then take a break and repeat for another 3 min.
Fast footwork drill	Repeat 7 times.
On the move drill	Perform 10 times, rest for 5 seconds and repeat 15 times.
Ladder drill	Perform for 3 min.
Cool-down	Hamstring and calf stretch (20-30 sec each leg); outward and inward shoulder stretch (20-30 sec each shoulder); and lying knee to chest (20 sec each leg)

Advanced Ultimate Form and Footwork Workout

The advanced form and footwork workout in figure 6.12 is right for you if you want to take your form and footwork skills to the highest levels. By super-boosting your stamina during a sweat-pouring workout that focuses on the execution of calorie-burning drills, you will master the skills needed to perform excellent boxing movements and get 100 percent confident in footwork and balance.

FIGURE 6.12   Advanced Ultimate Form and Footwork Workout

Warm-up	Perform the basic warm-up, intermediate warm-up or advanced warm-up from round 5.
Movements	Practise the forward and backward movement for 1 min followed by 1 min of shuffling movements.
Combination drill	Perform for 3 min; then take a break and repeat for another 3 min.
Fast footwork drill	Repeat 5 times.
On the move drill	Perform 10 times, rest for 5 seconds and repeat 15 times.
Ladder drill	Perform for 3 min.
Footwork clock drill	Perform for 4 to 6 min.
Cool-down	Hamstring and calf stretch (20-30 sec each leg); outward and inward shoulder stretch (20-30 sec each shoulder); and lying knee to chest (20 sec each leg)

In this round you learned your first set of boxing skills and drills and have now completed the first part of your journey to getting fitter with the fun boxing techniques used in the Total Knockout Fitness programme. It cannot be stressed enough that the way to a solid performance in boxing and boxing for fitness is getting the basics right first! Practising and mastering stance, guard and footwork will give you a head start and allow you to move on to learning how to punch your way to fitness and achieve great results.

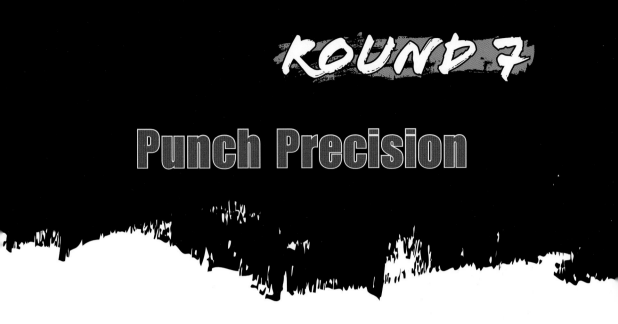

ROUND 7

Punch Precision

In this round we introduce you to simple and effective punching methods you can use to box your way to a better body. You've already learned the Total Knockout Fitness stance, guard and footwork techniques and safe ways to prepare your body for a great workout with a fun warm-up. You now have all the tools and know-how you need to learn to throw a punch with precision and power and take your skills and workouts to the next level.

The punch, a blow with the fist, is the only attack technique used in boxing. So what is the punch, what exercises can make it more powerful and how can you develop and improve your punching skills? This round answers these questions and provides a breakdown of several punch techniques: the jab, the cross, the hook and the uppercut. You will learn how to execute each of these punches, how to use specific exercises to master the techniques applied in the punching process and how to combine punches to create a super-effective upper-body routine to get you a step closer to your knockout physique. From basic, simple technique drills to more advanced, challenging skills training, you will be taken on a tour of boxing's core punch foundation.

Punch Basics

The Total Knockout Fitness workout routines include the jab, cross, hook and uppercut. If carried out frequently and correctly, these workouts will result in visible changes to your body and positive changes to your health and fitness. Once you have mastered the four boxing punches, you will be able to integrate them into the Total Knockout Fitness total-body workouts featured in round 8, fusing stress-busting, calorie-burning punch combinations with super-fast footwork skills and drills. This is your fast track to a fitter body and more balanced mind.

Each of the four punches in the Total Knockout Fitness programme has a specific use, technique, benefit and outcome. In competition, professional boxers aim to apply each of these punches at the right time to counter their opponents' attacks and try to hit their opponents with the right punch to achieve a knockout or score points for applying good technique. However, in the no-contact Total Knockout Fitness programme, the jab is used to develop arm muscles; the cross, to add flexibility to the torso; and the hook and the uppercut, to develop strength and definition in the upper body. Each of the punches improves the strength, flexibility and endurance of specific muscle groups to help you achieve a great, overall workout.

Technique must always take precedence over the application of force in a training programme. This promotes correct body alignment and optimum body position to generate force effectively. Because, generally, good technique reduces the wear and tear on a joint and dissipates the force evenly through the joint, keep your technique tight and correct at all times. The following points are also important to bear in mind when going through the punch combinations and exercises in this round:

✔ Remember that the basic techniques learned in the preliminary stages, including the guard and stance, are an important foundation for complex punching combinations. Keep practising these movements throughout your journey to develop great punching technique and power.

✔ Remember that you are only as strong as the planes of motion you work in. Make sure that your body positions, your arm and leg movements and the involvement of your back, legs and shoulders are correct.

✔ Always start slowly with the movement patterns.

✔ Hold the correct stance position between punches.

Following are some general, brief details and tips on the mechanics of punching, including how power is generated when punching a straight punch, how acceleration is achieved and what happens after the punch has been performed.

✔ The power of a punch comes from the ball of the foot; the energy transfers through the core as the trunk rotates around the central axis. The body fires the relaxed arm to the target in a straight line in the case of a cross or a jab, in a circular fashion in the case of a hook or up from the guard position in the case of an uppercut.

It is important that your arms remain relaxed. Start with your arms by your sides, feel the relaxation and then put your hands up. Gradually increase the speed of your punches while maintaining the relaxed feeling. Never forget to maintain your guard!

✔ The arm remains relaxed and transmits the force from the body. It accelerates with a final snap, the wrist turns and the palm faces the floor.

✔ After the punch, the fist retracts along the same path back to the guard position.

✔ The nonpunching hand remains in the guard position throughout.

Preparing for Punches

Preparing to deliver correct and safe punches will keep you safe during your boxing workouts and allow you to get the most out of your punch combinations as your accuracy improves. This section discusses some important points to remember before learning the various punch techniques.

Treat the Body as a Unit

Treating the body as a unit is a foundation of the Total Knockout Fitness programme. By keeping your body relaxed throughout your workout, you will avoid the temptation to perform unnatural movements too quickly and with a force your body cannot deal with. Although we discuss isolated body parts in this book, the whole body has to be synchronised when executing boxing techniques so that you use natural movements while working to improve your timing, speed and accuracy.

When executing punches, make sure that all movement starts at the ground level. Push off from the balls of your feet as the energy moves up through your body (hip and shoulder) and into the knuckles and onto the target. The body is one system; after movement starts in one part, it naturally flows to different parts, which has an energising effect, producing more motion. This smooth flow of natural movement results in a great, solid punching performance.

This round will help you get accustomed to the natural movement of your body when performing punches and boxing movements. By learning to throw your body weight from one side to the other, you will discover how to put your entire weight into your punches to maximise impact. Using your whole body in this way tones and shapes various body parts, increases muscle strength and enhances joint flexibility.

Punch Your Body Weight

One of the main goals of the Total Knockout Fitness programme is to punch with your whole body weight. Taking time to learn how to get the key punches flowing correctly with good movement and timing will help with the rest of the movements you will learn as the book progresses.

Stay Relaxed

Take a deep breath before you start your punches. You may feel slightly tense about learning these punches and performing high-speed combinations, especially if you are new to Total Knockout Fitness. Take your time, breathe in and out a few times and relax your whole body.

To get your body relaxed and in the right state to throw punches, try the swinging arms exercise. Relax your arms, let them hang down by your sides, soften your knees and stand with 70 percent of your weight on the balls of your feet. Swing from side to side, allowing your arms to be free; turn your body from left to right so that your arms swing out horizontally. Do not control your arms; get used to the movement, pushing from one foot and then the other, noticing how your torso turns from side to side and the natural movement of your hips, torso and arms swinging. Perform this for one minute. This should take away the edge you may be feeling as you step up to throwing punches. It is also an additional way to warm up your arms, shoulders and torso.

If at any time you feel overwhelmed by the techniques, stop for a minute, refocus and return to the techniques you already mastered. For example, if you have difficulty getting a technique right, leave it for a minute and practise the stance and guard. When you have cleared your mind and feel ready, go back to the punch technique and take it step by step, going through each step slowly.

Learn the Basics

When learning a punch, study the basics first and make sure you understand the techniques inside out. Applying the correct techniques for guard, stance and punches builds muscle endurance and overall fitness. Performing

Three Tips for Every Punch

To add that bit of edge to your punch and raise the speed and accuracy bar for your punching skills, follow these tips:

1. Breathe through your nose and not your mouth when throwing a punch. Breathing through your nose increases the quality of the punch because of the force with which you exhale.

2. Exhale when you throw the punch and inhale when you retract your arm and resume the guard position. Exhaling when throwing a punch adds to the force of the punch; inhaling as you retract the punch replenishes your oxygen supply.

3. Always use your free arm, the arm you are not throwing a punch with, to protect your body and head.

punches correctly builds muscle around the connective tissue in the wrists, elbows and shoulders, which improves your posture and strengthens and tones the muscles around your rib cage and spine. A punch executed correctly not only increases the intensity of your workout, but also adds to the fun of boxing for fitness.

With each new punch, read through the background information, when it is used, how to perform it correctly and how to integrate it into a simple boxing combination. This round teaches you how to throw the four main punches properly and safely, giving you advice and tips that will help you develop and maintain a slick repertoire of punches and combinations as you progress on your journey to a fitter body.

Take Breaks

As you go through the various techniques and exercises in this round, always remember the importance of taking breaks between learning new techniques. Throw the required single punches or combinations, and then stop and reflect on how you feel when you are throwing the punches. Ask yourself how accurate your punches were and whether your knuckles hit the target with enough speed and power. Then think of how you can improve the next time you throw the same punch or combination. Only then should you learn a new technique.

Practice Makes Perfect

There is no such thing as overpractising in Total Knockout Fitness. If you want to get your basics right, master the boxing combinations and realise the physical and emotional benefits of this programme, give it your all, learn thoroughly and practise until you can perform the techniques in your sleep. The Total Knockout Fitness programme has proven to thousands of enthusiasts across the world that with lots of practice you can achieve really great outcomes for your body, mind and fitness level. So don't be shy; get those punches (and sweat pearls) flowing if you too want to feel and look great after a good, honest workout.

At the same time, don't overthink. Once you have tried the techniques step by step, repeat them in slow motion a few times. When you have the hang of it, accelerate the speed of the punch. As your technique tightens and you don't have to consciously think of each step to get the punch right, your confidence will grow and you will begin to throw effective punches. Just be patient and thorough when you first start with a new technique. Make sure you've got it completely right, and then practise, practise, practise until you've mastered it and feel you can throw jabs, crosses, uppercuts and hooks effortlessly.

Stay Safe

To protect your wrists, shoulders and lower spine, adopt the correct stance and guard before executing a punch. This will protect your body when performing punches. For example, maintaining the correct stance will lower the risk of injury to your lower spine when rotating to throw a cross. Remember to perform your movement from the ground up, applying correct stance, guard and hook techniques, and pay great attention to accuracy as you throw a punch towards your target.

Total Knockout Fitness Punches

This section outlines the punches used in this programme. You will learn how to throw the jab, cross, hook and uppercut and some great exercises to make them the calorie-burning tools you want them to be. Let's get started!

Range Finder

A range finder is a punch, generally a jab, thrown to check the distance between yourself and your target. For training purposes this is done in a stationary position; in sparring and boxing it is thrown on the move. Finding range means extending your arm in a punch format to check the distance between you and your opponent or a target to establish a safe and appropriate distance.

The jab is the range finder punch. If you are right-handed, use your left hand as a range finder; if you are left-handed, use your right hand as a range finder. On average, you will throw three jabs to one cross.

Jab

The jab is delivered with the arm that is above the lead foot, or the arm nearer the target. This means that if your left foot is the lead foot, you will deliver a jab with your left arm, and if your right foot is the lead foot, you will deliver a jab with your right arm. In boxing, the jab is a quick and explosive punch mostly used to distract the opponent, keep distance, set up for a punch combination and defend from an opponent's attacks. It is also used to build up the attack and keep the opponent guessing where the boxer is going to punch. You could say that a boxer with no jab is like a basketball player who can't dribble.

In boxing, just as in any other sport or activity, it is vital to start from the ground and work your way up step by step and bit by bit. A solid jab is the foundation of good punching technique that will get you fit and in shape. Getting the jab technique right and using the Total Knockout Fitness exercises featured in this round (which include both single and combination punching) will allow you to move on to trickier boxing for fitness skills and ultimately advance your fitness level.

If you are right-handed, to execute the jab, start from the midlevel guard and upright stance position (see figure 7.1a). Keep your chin down to avoid holding your head too high. Push down and twist off the ball of your left foot to start the movement. With your lead hand, extend your arm almost fully and twist your arm in a corkscrew motion just before completion. This means that halfway through throwing the punch forwards, your forearm rotates in the last quarter of the movement so that your thumb is facing the floor when the punch is completed (see figure 7.1b). At the contact point, make sure your elbow is still soft and that you your shoulders are relaxed. The rotation of the forearm will give you the snap you need for a good punch. The nonpunching hand stays in guard position throughout. After making contact, quickly return to the starting position.

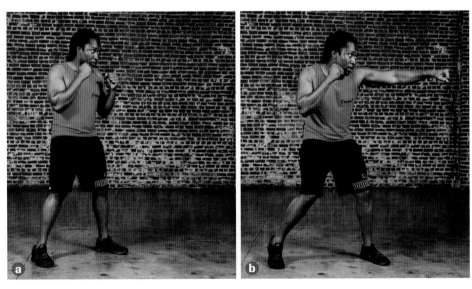

FIGURE 7.1 The jab.

MULTIPLE JABS

In boxing, in addition to being a range finding punch, the jab is a good defensive punch. In fitness, it is a good setup punch for the cross and improves the strength and endurance of the shoulder muscles. If you are not a professional boxer, throwing the jab three times to one cross is a great way to build strength in your weaker arm. It builds endurance and strength and energizes the neuropathways and motor skills in that arm. Using your weaker arm to jab three times to every jab with your preferred arm will increase the signals sent from the brain through the neuropathways to the weaker arm, making it more active. As a result, you may find that everyday activities (e.g., picking up shopping bags) carried out with your weaker arm are much easier. Increasing strength in your weaker arm can also help balance your body so that it is not so one-sided.

To throw multiple jabs, begin in the upright stance and midlevel guard position. Start throwing jabs, gradually building up your speed. Focus on getting a sharp, clean punch, finish and come back to the stance and guard position, wait two seconds and then throw the punch again.

Note that the nonpunching hand is on guard at all times. Try throwing three jabs at one time; then throw three more jabs at a faster speed, and then five jabs (this 3-3-5 sequence is a typical recurring training method in the Total Knockout Fitness programme). Practise multiple jabs as prescribed here until you feel confident throwing a jab using the correct technique.

JAB TWIST

The jab twist builds endurance in the forearms and triceps and can increase joint stability by strengthening the elbow and shoulder joints. Start in the mid-level guard and upright stance position. Try the jab technique with a twist by pushing through from the ball of the foot, twisting, and rotating through to the hips, shoulder and fist. This is a movement pattern through which the energy is transferred from the ground up as the body rotates around the central axis. You should be able to feel how this twist, or snap, improves your punch power when throwing a jab. Try to feel your shoulder being thrust into the punch. Remember whipping a towel at your friends when you were a kid? The jab is just like that towel. Always remember that you are aiming for a quick, straight and precise jab; this snap will give you the extra bit to perfect your technique. See figure 7.2 for an example of the jab twist.

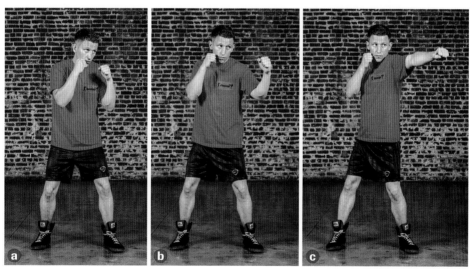

FIGURE 7.2   Jab twist.

JAB AT DIFFERENT HEIGHTS

The jab at different heights consists of high, medium and low punching and builds the glutes, hamstrings and quadriceps and improves coordination. Throw a jab with your knuckles in line with your eyes; then throw a midpunch, which is 5 centimetres (2 in.) lower than your shoulder and, finally, squat down 7 to 10 centimetres (3 to 4 in.) on your legs and throw the jab from this position. Repeat nine times, stopping after each set of punches, and focus on the accuracy, twist and speed of the punch. Rest three seconds between sets. See figure 7.3 for an example of the jab at different heights.

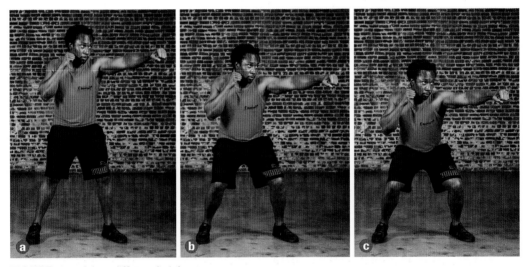

FIGURE 7.3   Jab at different heights.

Cross

The cross is a direct punch delivered with the rear hand. It is considered a power punch: The fist crosses in front of the body and in front of the lead arm; power is generated through the rotation of the hips while the rear foot is at a 45-degree angle to the body.

In the professional boxing world, many boxers use the cross as a counterpunch to a jab, aiming for the opponent's head, as a counter to a cross aimed at the body or to set up to throwing a hook. In the Total Knockout Fitness programme and in the very traditional, classic punch combination, the cross can also follow a jab, resulting in the simple 'one-two combination' (one standing for cross, two standing for jab). The cross generates more power than the jab because the hand travels a greater distance and therefore generates more speed and momentum on its way to the target. The position of the back leg makes it easy to push off and add more body weight to the punch, which creates more speed, force and power.

If you are right-handed, to execute the cross, start in the midlevel guard and upright stance position (see figure 7.4a); 70 percent of your weight should be on your balls of your feet. The rear foot is turned 45 degrees away from the body as always. The shoulders are in line with the target (this is called the power line) offering protection for the right side of your jaw. Your dominant fist rests beneath your chin because the movement of your hand should start from your chin. Throw your rear hand from the chin, crossing your body and propelling your hand towards the target in a straight line directly from your face to the target (see figure 7.4b), then return to midlevel guard (see figure 7.4c). The left hand remains at midlevel guard throughout this movement.

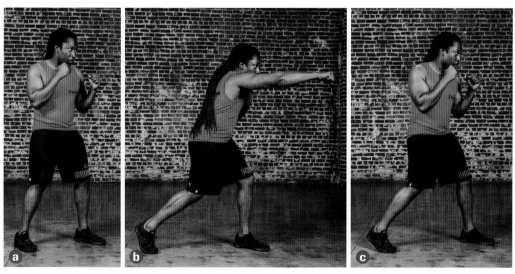

FIGURE 7.4 The cross.

The power of the cross is generated by the body rotation and the sudden weight transfer during the movement. To generate additional power, you can add a half step forwards with the rear foot to your movement. To gain even more power, you can rotate the torso and hips anticlockwise and transfer your weight from the rear to the lead foot as you throw the cross. Retract your lead hand and tuck it against your face to protect the inside of your chin. After you have thrown the cross, retract your hand quickly and maintain the midlevel guard and upright stance position.

Punch Blast

In the upright stance and midlevel guard position, pay attention to maintaining your triangular base and applying good rotation around your body's central axis when executing continuous punching. Your body, especially your shoulders, should be relaxed; avoid clenching your fists too tightly. The power is transferred from the ground up to ensure good rotation from the hips around your body's central axis. Remember to keep the nonpunching hand in guard position to protect the jaw and to keep the elbow tucked into the ribs.

If possible, stand in front of a mirror, at least 25 centimetres (10 in.) away, and aim for your chin in the reflection. Jab and cross punches go straight to the centre of the chin, and hooks go to either side (the left hook lands on the left side and the right hook lands on the right side).

> Round 1: Jab-cross
> Round 2: Jab-cross-hook-cross (hook with the lead hand)
> Round 3: Jab-cross-duck-hook-hook

SINGLE CROSS WITH TECHNIQUE FOCUS

Facing a mirror, focus on the centre of your chin (you could mark this with a piece of tape on a wall if no mirror is available). Now, driving the power up from the ball of the rear foot and through the thighs, rotate the hips, torso and shoulders around your body's central axis and aim for the centre of the first two knuckles to align with the centre of your chin (in the mirror, or with the tape on the wall). Pay particular attention to performing the movements correctly. Start off slowly, and as the technique becomes fluid, increase the speed. See figure 7.5 for an example of the single cross with technique focus.

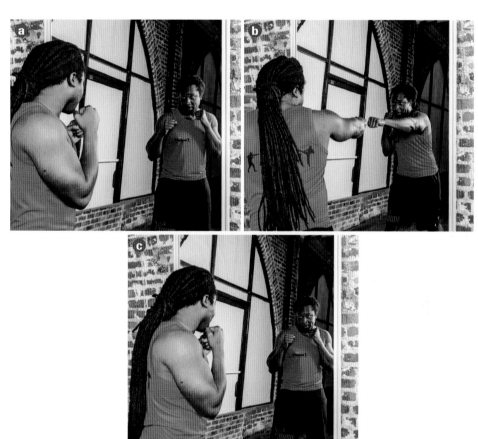

FIGURE 7.5 Single cross with technique focus.

Mirror Boxing

Mirror and shadowboxing drills offer a great preparation for a boxing-based workout by getting the muscles ready for the workout while also engaging and focusing the mind on the task at hand. They can also offer a cardiorespiratory workout depending on the intensity. Using a mirror allows you to check that you are using the correct techniques and make any adjustments required.

By fixing some tape to a mirror, you can mark some key points such as the central axis and the position of the elbows. You can also mark a cross at a specific target such as the centre of the chin to assist with teaching points and correct techniques.

If you are shadowboxing or boxing in front of a mirror:

1. Find a point to focus on and aim your punches at that point. In shadowboxing you are throwing punches at an imaginary point.

2. Picture your target (e.g., a specific point on a bag or a pad or whatever else you want it to be).

3. Aim the centre of the knuckles of your index and middle fingers to hit your chosen target.

4. Keep the same target for a while to get used to it and improve your accuracy.

If you have a mirror, practise the jab by focusing your shot on the centre of your chin. Do not stand too close to the mirror to avoid making contact. Focus on your two knuckles (again, the knuckles of the index and middle fingers) when throwing punches. Push and lunge forwards off the back leg and throw your jab, sliding your whole body forwards at the end of the movement and keeping your focus on this point at all times. Don't forget to exhale as you perform the punch and inhale on the retraction. This type of mirror training will improve your eye–hand coordination and accuracy.

CROSS WITH SPEED AND POWER FOCUS

This exercise is also ideally performed facing a mirror and focusing on the centre of your chin (you could mark this with a piece of tape on a wall if no mirror is available). Now, driving the power up from the ball of the rear foot and through the thighs, rotate the hips, torso and shoulders around your body's central axis and aim for the centre of the first two knuckles to align with the centre of the chin (in the mirror, or with the tape on the wall). Throw three crosses with maximum force; then take a five-second break to make any adjustments to your technique and check your stance.

CROSS COMBO TO THE HEAD AND BODY

Once again, use a mirror to focus on the centre of your chin as well as your solar plexus (where the ribs join just below the centre of the chest); if no mirror is available, mark these heights on a wall with tape. Now, driving the power up from the ball of the rear foot and through the thighs, rotate the hips, torso and shoulders around your body's central axis and aim for the centre of the first two knuckles to align with the centre of the chin. Immediately lower your bodyweight so your shoulders are aligned with the target, throw the cross to that target and return to midlevel guard and upright stance.

JAB-CROSS COMBINATION

Now that you have learned how to perform a real jab and an effective cross, you are ready to put your technique to the test with straight punch combinations and to practise your technique once more. Start with a jab, return to midlevel guard and stance position, follow up with a cross and return to midlevel guard and upright stance position. Repeat this three times with five-second breaks between sets. Then perform the combination again three times with another five-second break, followed by a set of five to finish this exercise.

Four Ways to Increase Your Punching Power

Following are four simple yet highly effective ways to add extra power to your punches.

1. *Don't arm punch.* Most novices and untrained fighters are guilty of arm punching, which means that they throw the punch with the arm without involving the torso and legs. Instead of using their legs, back and core muscles to add power and body weight to their punches, arm punchers rely on their often relatively weak shoulders and triceps to throw a punch. To increase punching power, avoid arm punching.

2. *Shift your weight.* Add that extra edge and power to your punches by shifting a percentage of your weight from one foot to the other. Briefly, get your body weight moving with the punch! Practising the transfer of weight from one foot to another while throwing a punch also increases your ability to string together a series of punches, which allows you to move on to our exciting boxing combinations.

3. *Step with the punch.* Stepping when you punch is a simple way to increase your punch power; it applies to all punches except uppercuts.

4. *Pivot with the punch.* Pivoting can significantly strengthen your punches. The pivoting movement starts with the unweighted foot and continues up your body. This puts more body mass behind the punch and hugely increases your power.

Hook

The hook, which involves turning the body to aim towards the side of the head or body of the opponent, is a powerful punch with knockout power in boxing. It is executed by turning the core muscles and back and swinging the arm, which is bent at an angle near or at 90 degrees, in a horizontal arc towards the opponent; it can be aimed at the head or at the body. The hook can be thrown by either the lead hand or the rear hand. In the Total Knockout Fitness programme, you will use a hook primarily with the lead hand.

There are three types of hooks: short-, mid- and long-range hooks; the choice depends on the distance from the opponent or target. The Total Knockout Fitness programme uses the long-range hook because you are positioned at a right angle, with shoulders horizontal, making it easier to throw. When throwing a hook, aim to execute it with precision and speed—a short, fast and direct punch provides the best results. In boxing, often the best time to throw a hook is after a right cross. This is reflected in the traditional combination of jab, right cross, left hook, which is a combination used in the Total Knockout Fitness programme. This is because throwing the right hand puts you in a perfect position to throw an effective left hook.

To execute the right hook, start in the upright stance and midlevel guard position. Turn your body in a snapping motion, shifting your body weight to the rear, which pivots the lead foot and torso in the direction of your punch. Think of it as a three-step process: first pivot the foot; then pivot the hips and then the hand in the direction of your punch. Bring your left arm from the side when throwing the left hook; bring your right arm from the side when throwing the right hook. Remember, when throwing punches, to keep your chin down near your leading shoulder and keep eyes focused on your target. When throwing the hook, always make sure your palms are facing inwards rather than towards the floor; this position is much safer and reduces the risk of injury to the wrist. Swing your lead fist horizontally towards your target, facing your palms inwards. Connect with your target with the first two knuckles. See figure 7.6 for an example of the hook.

Pivoting increases the power of the hook; however, proper arm swinging holds the key to this punch. When propelling the fist towards the target, your hand should be bent at an angle of around 90 degrees and you should transfer your entire body weight onto your rear foot to create that all-important power, precision and speed in your punch.

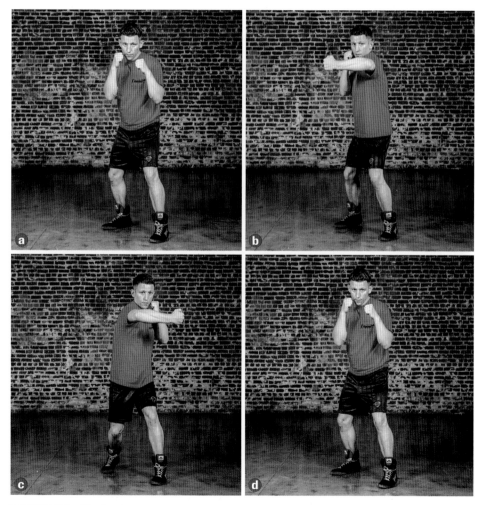

FIGURE 7.6 The hook.

SINGLE HOOK

First, adopt the upright stance and midlevel guard position with your feet shoulder-width apart. Take a natural step forwards with the lead foot, keeping the shoulders in line with the toes. Turn the rear foot out 45 degrees (this foot position forms a triangle, with both feet and the backside) and bend the knees. Raise your hands up above your head and bring your fingers down and place your thumbs over the outside of them to form a fist. Drop your elbows in to protect your ribs and position your fists in line with your jaw with your palms facing inwards. Tipping slightly forwards from your hips, place 70 percent of your body weight on the balls of your feet. Drive the force from the ball of the lead foot up through a pivot motion in the legs and hips as you raise the elbow of your punching arm. Throw three single hooks and then take a five-second break to double-check your technique. Check that your feet are in the correct triangular stance and that your elbow is bent to 90 degrees as you drive the hip through. Then, throw three more single hooks and take another five-second break to check your technique again. Now throw five more single hooks with your lead hand, and then switch to the rear hand. See figure 7.7 for an example of the single hook.

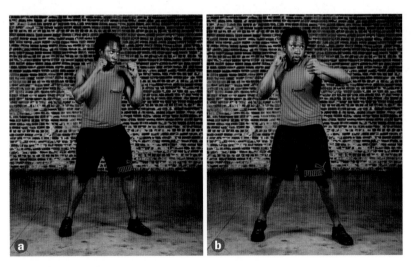

FIGURE 7.7   Single hook.

HOOK ROTATION

To practise and perfect the hook, start by raising both elbows to 90 degrees and bring your fists together. With knuckles touching in front of your chin, begin to rotate around the central axis as your force drives from the ball of the lead foot up in a pivot motion through the legs, hips and shoulders. See figure 7.8 for an example of a hook rotation.

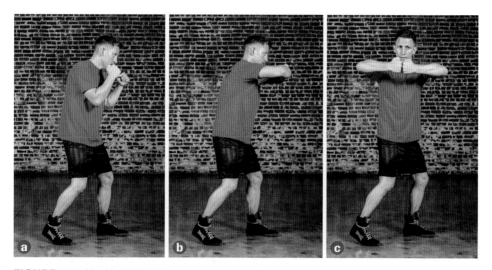

FIGURE 7.8 Hook rotation.

FOUR-PUNCH HOOK COMBO

From the upright stance and midlevel guard position, throw a four-punch hook combination as follows: lead hook, rear hook, lead hook, rear hook. Notice again the circular motion as you rotate your hips and shoulders around the centre of your body. Be sure to return the nonpunching hand to the guard position. See figure 7.9 for an example of the four-punch hook combo.

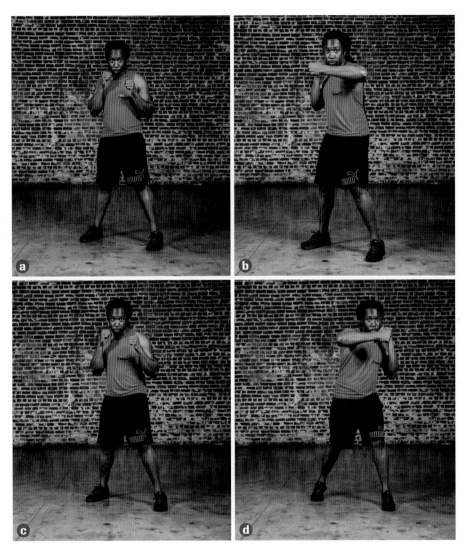

FIGURE 7.9 Four-punch hook combo.

Visualise a Point

To create faster and more powerful punches, have a go at the following visualisation exercise.

1. At the start of the visualisation, make sure you are in a relaxed state, nice and warm. A good way to do this is to think of a time in which you were very focused and motivated to take action (e.g., another sporting activity, a competition). Recall the images you were seeing at that time, any sounds that may have been associated with those images and any feelings you were having. Then focus on a specific point (a centre point is usually best) on a focus pad or bag in front of you, and throw your combinations to either side of it. If you do not have a physical target, simply imagine one and aim for the point you have chosen (e.g., an imaginary point or the stitching of a pad or bag). You could also focus on a spot on the wall. Always keep a safe distance from a physical target to avoid injuring your wrists or fists.

2. Visualise your chosen point precisely and imagine yourself hitting that point perfectly with two knuckles every time you throw a punch.

3. When throwing your punch at your target, make sure you are relaxed and in a natural position, leaning slightly forwards from the hips and with soft knees.

Do this visualisation technique several times and really get into the combinations. Then practise for two to five minutes according to your fitness level.

Uppercut

The uppercut is often praised as a brilliant knockout punch aimed at the opponent's chin. Although you can generate a good amount of power for most punches, the cross and uppercut are generally considered power punches because of the dropping of the knees to a lower level and the slight bending of the knees, which generates force. Usually, the uppercut starts slightly underneath the chest, allowing the hand to be propelled vertically in a swift, fast hook-shaped movement towards the opponent's face or body or a visualised target. In traditional boxing, the uppercut is often thrown after the jab, but of course it can appear at the start or finish of any boxing combination. Uppercuts can be thrown with either hand. A boxer can choose between short-, medium- and long-range uppercuts depending on the distance from the opponent. The Total Knockout Fitness programme mainly uses the long-range uppercut for extra safety and to reduce the risk of injury.

In the professional boxing environment, uppercuts are most effective when thrown at close range, where they can cause the most damage to the opponent (the goal of any boxer). A boxer who throws an uppercut from too far away would probably miss the opponent's chin. Moreover, the opponent at a distance would probably detect the uppercut and thus have an opportunity to counter with a straight punch. Because it is a slightly more advanced punch, the uppercut is a great addition to your Total Knockout Fitness repertoire because it works more areas of your body, strengthens the muscles in your arms and makes your workout more fun.

To execute the uppercut with the lead hand, start in the upright stance and midlevel guard position. Hold your arms close to your body, and keep your rear hand up by your chin to protect your head. With your feet shoulder-width apart, step forwards with the lead leg, keeping your feet in line with your shoulders (see figure 7.10*a*). Now take the back foot out 45 degrees, make sure you are leaning slightly forwards from the hips, bend the knees and drop down slightly (see figure 7.10*b*). With your eyes always on the target, make a U shape with your head, which results in a circular movement in your body (see figure 7.10*c*). Twist your body inwards and push up by rotating your hips forwards and pushing up from the ball of the back (right) foot. Throw the left fist up towards the target (see figure 7.10*d*). The left arm always stays close to the body and moves upwards in a semicircle. The U moves to the left as you throw your hand at the same time, releasing it when you get to the top of the U. While performing this movement, make sure that the left side of the back and the left shoulder follow through with the rotation of the hips. Keep the palm facing inwards at all times. At the finishing position, the hips should be squared to the front, back in the guard position.

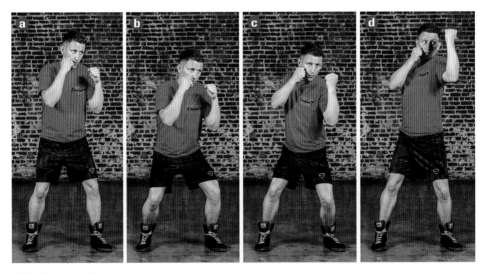

FIGURE 7.10   The uppercut.

CORKSCREW

Settle your body weight down into your thighs and butt and drive up from the floor in a corkscrew motion rotating the hip and torso and keeping the hands in the guard position. The purpose of this exercise is to create maximum force and flow through the body. See figure 7.11 for an example of the corkscrew.

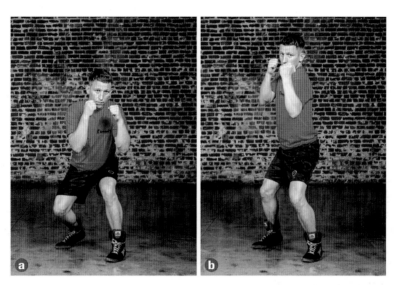

FIGURE 7.11 Corkscrew.

UPPERCUT DRILL

Settle your body weight down into the thighs and butt and drive up from the floor in a corkscrew motion rotating the hip and torso and keeping the hands in the guard position. Follow the guidance on how to perform a safe and correct uppercut and this time, as you throw the uppercut, turn the wrist so the palm faces you and driving the fist up towards the target until it is 2.5 to 5 centimetres (1 or 2 in.) from the target at the end of the movement. See figure 7.12 for an example of the uppercut drill.

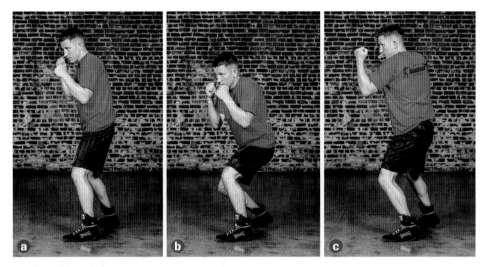

FIGURE 7.12 Uppercut drill.

FOUR UPPERCUTS DRILL

Settle your body weight down into the thighs and butt and drive up from the floor in a corkscrew motion rotating the hip and torso and keeping the hands in the guard position. Follow the steps in in the corkscrew drill and this time add four uppercuts by turning the wrist so the palm faces you and driving the fist up towards the target until you are within 2.5 to 5 centimetres (1 or 2 in.) of the target at the end of the movement. See figure 7.13 for an example of the four uppercuts drill.

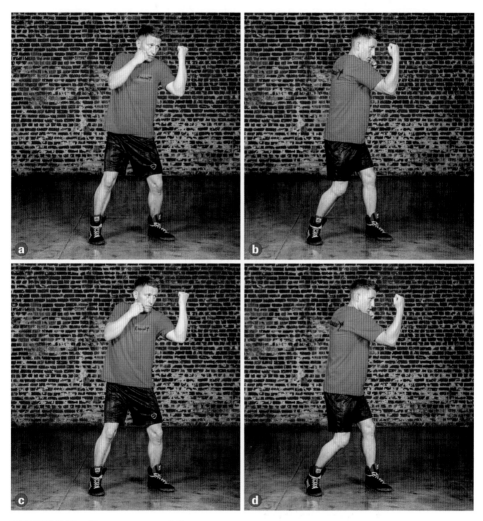

FIGURE 7.13 Four uppercuts drill.

Increase the power of your punches with these nonequipment exercises.

Squat Punch

The squat punch tones the legs and bum while stimulating the metabolism. Begin in the upright stance and midlevel guard position. Bending from the knees, settle your body weight down to load your legs and bottom (see figure 7.14a). Drive up through the balls of your feet and throw a punch or punch combination (see figure 7.14b).

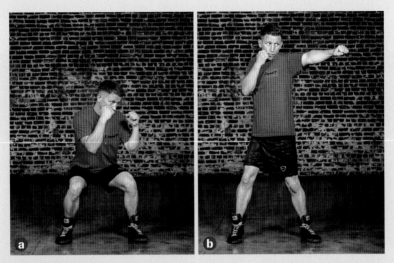

FIGURE 7.14   Squat punch.

Twist Jump and Punch

The twist jump and punch is a fun, dynamic exercise that is guaranteed to strengthen and tone the tummy while burning fat fast! Begin in the upright stance and midlevel guard position paying attention to the target where you will land your punches. Throw a jab-cross-jab-cross combination, driving from the balls of your feet until you leave the floor. Twist from your core and rotate 180 degrees so that you land in a perfect Total Knockout Fitness stance facing in the opposite direction and repeat.

Squat Jump Shuffle

The squat jump shuffle is an opportunity to challenge your reflexes and test your skills. Remember the 2-2-2-2 pattern footwork pattern that you mastered during the basic and intermediate workout routines.

Perform a shuffle and then a jab-cross-jab-cross combination, followed by a squat punch (see figure 7.14, a and b) at the end of each movement so that you perform the following patterns:

> Two forward shuffles, a jab-cross-jab-cross combination and a squat punch
> Two backward shuffles, a jab-cross-jab-cross combination and a squat punch
> Two left shuffles, a jab-cross-jab-cross combination and a squat punch
> Two right shuffles, a jab-cross-jab-cross combination and a squat punch

Remember to focus on the correct movement and maintain that all-important base so you are using your body efficiently!

Total Knockout Fitness Ultimate Upper-Body Workout

Now that you have learned techniques and tools for throwing the four main punches, try the following traditional combination in figure 7.15 for a great upper-body workout.

Do the following punches 20 times each for three sets with a one-minute rest between sets.

FIGURE 7.15   Ultimate Upper-Body Workout

Warm-up	Perform the basic warm-up, intermediate warm-up or advanced warm-up from round 5.		
Warm-up	**Reps**	**Sets**	**Rest**
Right jab	20	3	1 min
Left hook	20	3	1 min
Left jab	20	3	1 min
Right uppercut	20	3	1 min
Left hook	20	3	1 min
Right cross	20	3	1 min
Cool-down	Hamstring and calf stretch (20-30 sec each leg); outward and inward shoulder stretch (20-30 sec each shoulder); and lying knee to chest (20 sec each leg)		

Now that you are familiar with the four main punches in boxing, you will soon master them and be able to integrate them into an effective upper-body routine to help you achieve your goal, whether you want to lose weight, get fitter, get stronger, become more flexible or simply enjoy the fun of boxing for a fitness training routine. The next round explores tips and tricks for throwing your super-punches while on the move. Get ready to add some great endurance and cardiorespiratory benefits to your fitness repertoire.

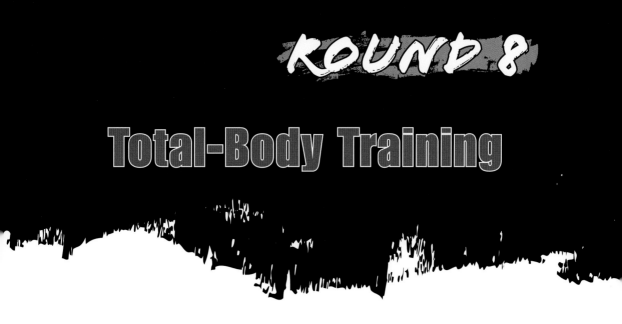

ROUND 8

Total-Body Training

In this round you will combine the skills you have acquired over the course of your Total Knockout Fitness journey from round 1 to round 7. You will learn fun ways to combine super-fast footwork drills with more advanced punch combinations. The goal is to provide you with a variety of techniques so you can create a total-body workout that suits your requirements and ability levels and helps you reach your fitness and health goals. The exercises and punch combinations outlined here will increase your stamina and encourage you to work faster, harder and with more focus. You will further perfect your footwork skills, improve your punching technique and learn how to combine these two elements with increasing ease and confidence.

After learning what total-body training means, you will learn how to prepare for this type of intense training and tools you can apply to achieve maximum benefits for your body and mind. You will also build on the basics of footwork discussed in round 6 and develop more advanced footwork techniques by integrating dynamic horizontal and lateral movements while throwing punches. At the end of this round are Total Knockout Fitness total-body routines that range from simple to advanced; choose the one that fits your body and level of fitness.

What Is Total-Body Training?

In the Total Knockout Fitness programme, total-body training is training that uses all the major muscle groups in a calorie-busting upper- and lower-body workout that incorporates forward, backward and side-to-side movements with punch combinations. Your body benefits all over, from strengthening your arms, legs and shoulders to toning your abdomen and glutes from the inside out. Total-body training burns a lot of calories and raises the heart rate to boost cardiorespiratory fitness. The following sections outline the benefits of Total Knockout Fitness total-body training.

Increase Fitness Level

Total-body training is a super-effective way to increase your overall fitness, strength and flexibility while fine-tuning your exercise and punching techniques. The total-body workout routines featured in this book combine boxing for fitness skills and drills with exercises that work the entire body as a functional unit, allowing you to release stress and increase your focus and overall sense of well-being.

Reduce Stress Level

Total Knockout Fitness total-body training offers great benefits to the mind by stimulating, energising and de-stressing your entire body. Performing any type of safe exercise distracts your mind from things that stress or worry you. Your stress level will decrease as you focus on the job at hand: punching your way to a fitter, healthier body.

Energise Your Body

Combining footwork and punching drills in regular exercise routines will improve the way you feel about yourself. You may find that you have much more energy and feel better and healthier. Moving around while throwing punch combinations also raises your heart rate, which brings fresh oxygen to your body and activates your muscles.

Footwork Refresher

Before you begin learning the total-body exercises and routines outlined in this round, make sure you are confident in applying the footwork skills you learned in round 6 and that you can perform footwork drills with quick, clean movements. Here is a mini-review of footwork to refresh your memory about the main things to remember (for more detailed information, refer back to round 6):

> Make sure that 70 percent of your weight is on the balls of your feet.

> Make a short, sliding movement with light contact on the floor; then accelerate your movements while trying to minimise upper-body movement. Your body weight should be equally balanced through both legs until the point of impact.

> Lean slightly forwards from the hips about 5 centimetres (2 in.) or so.

> When you are moving forwards, the push comes from the back foot. The front foot moves first and the back foot follows.

> When you are moving backwards, the back foot moves first and the front foot follows the same distance.

> Do not take big steps. Keep them short.

Total-Body Exercises

Now it is time to combine the skills you learned over the last rounds into total-body exercises. Before you do this, however, be sure you have mastered the stance and guard position. Also, you need to have the techniques for punches and combinations completely locked down so you can easily integrate them into the total-body training routines. Round 7 outlined all of the punch techniques and their various combinations; if you need to refresh your memory and practise them some more, now is the time. Once you are confident with all of the techniques, it is time to get moving.

A lateral side stretch is just the thing to prepare your body for moving forwards, backwards and laterally. To do this, stand with your feet shoulder-width apart. Reach your arms over your head and stretch up right through your fingertips, lengthening your whole body. Keep your abdominal muscles tight and your chest straight and open. Now stretch over to the left, lengthening the right side of your upper body. You should feel the stretch through your ribs and back. As you rise, inhale. Then stretch up and over to the right, lengthening the left side of your body. Hold both positions for 30 seconds.

Following is a set of simple exercises that will teach you the basics of total-body training.

When moving forwards and backwards, remember that the front foot takes you forwards and the back foot takes you backwards. You drive from the opposite foot so when moving forwards, for example, you push through the floor with the back foot.

MOVING AND SHIFTING

The main component of this exercise is moving forwards and backwards by sliding your feet smoothly and shifting your body weight. This exercise will help you move faster and with more power while defining your leg muscles and firming your bottom.

Start in the upright stance and midlevel guard position (see figure 8.1*a*). Keep your upper body in guard position while moving forwards one step, using your front leg first and letting your back leg follow. When you step forwards, push off the ball of your back foot and slide forwards (see figure 8.1*b*). This movement can also be described as loading your back leg because you drop down a few centimetres (an inch or so) with slightly more bent knees and shift your body weight towards your back leg. Repeat this five times until you have completed five steps. Then do the same backwards until you reach your starting point. Repeat this exercise three times in both directions, increasing the speed of your legs with each repetition.

While doing this exercise, imagine that you are throwing a straight punch after each step, but don't actually throw punches. Performing this exercise without actually throwing a punch allows you to concentrate solely on your footwork, focusing on moving forwards and backwards in clean, smooth, swift movements. It will also improve your ability to keep your balance when moving around.

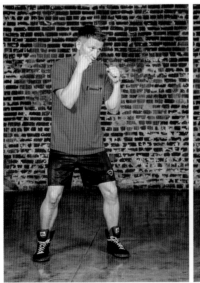 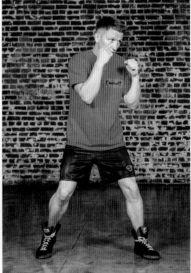

FIGURE 8.1 Moving and shifting forwards.

MOVING AND SHIFTING WITH PUNCHES

This exercise integrates punching techniques with footwork skills, allowing you to practise them both and simulate a real boxing experience. This movement can also be described as loading your back leg because you drop down an inch (2.5 cm or so) with slightly bent knees and shift your body weight towards your back leg. Start in the upright stance and midlevel guard position. Stay in this position while moving forwards one step, using your lead leg first and then your back leg. Lower your back leg just as you move forwards, pushing off the ball of your foot and sliding forwards. After each step, throw a jab-cross-jab-cross punch combination following the techniques detailed in round 7 (as you progress, you can try throwing a hook-cross-hook-cross combination). When moving, always keep your eyes focused on the target of your punches.

Repeat this exercise five times until you have completed five steps; then do the same backwards until you reach your starting point. Repeat this exercise three times to get used to the movement of sliding forwards with speed and power while throwing punch combinations correctly. Always remember that your goal is to master footwork so you can move quickly, keep your balance and burn more calories; this can only happen when you move with speed and power at all times. Performing this exercise in front of a mirror can hugely improve your performance because you can check and improve your technique and aim the knuckles of your index and middle finger at a focus point in the mirror.

MOVING SIDE TO SIDE

This exercise is great for improving your footwork and balance and increasing the speed of your feet, which will ultimately get you sweating and help to burn more calories. Start in the upright stance and midlevel guard position (see figure 8.2*a*). Stay in this position while moving to the left one step, using your lead leg first and then your back leg (see figure 8.2*b*). This is done by pushing off the ball of your back foot, sliding your lead foot to the left and following an equal distance with the back foot. Shift your bodyweight onto your back leg just as you move forwards, pushing off the ball of your rear foot and sliding forwards. Remember, when moving to the right, to push off with your left foot in a lateral direction, move your right foot first and follow an equal distance with your left. When moving to the left, push off with your right foot in a lateral direction move your left foot first and follow an equal distance with your right. After each step, throw a jab-cross-jab-cross punch combination following the techniques detailed in round 7. When moving, always keep your eyes focused on the target of your punches.

Repeat this exercise five times until you have completed five steps; then do the same in the opposite direction until you reach your starting point. As your confidence in moving laterally grows, you can increase the speed of your legs. Always make sure the quality of your movements is high and that you are able to move smoothly and quickly.

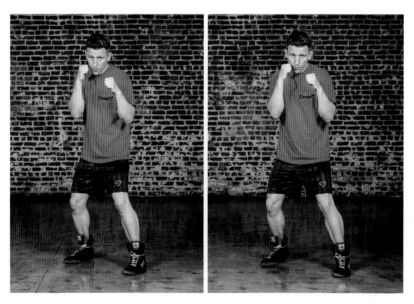

FIGURE 8.2 Moving to the side.

15-Minute Express Total-Body Workouts

The Total Knockout Fitness 15-minute express total-body training workouts have three key elements: warm-up, main session and cool-down. Before attempting these routines, make sure you have mastered the form and footwork techniques in round 6 and the punching skills in round 7. This is important not only to ensure your safety but also to make sure you get the full benefits from your workout.

Following are three 15-minute express workouts: basic, intermediate and advanced. There is something fun here for every ability and fitness level.

Basic 15-Minute Express Workout

The basic 15-minute express workout in figure 8.3 provides a solid base for all Total Knockout Fitness boxing for fitness techniques and exercises. This short workout tones and strengthens the whole body while raising your awareness of your body and your own natural movement patterns. It combines Total Knockout Fitness boxing techniques with a mental focus to address the mind–body connection and provide the holistic benefits of stress relief and improved focus.

FIGURE 8.3   Basic 15-Minute Express Total-Body Workout

Warm-up	Perform the basic warm-up, intermediate warm-up or advanced warm-up from round 5.			
Main session	Stance and guard: Get in the stance and guard, 5 sec on, 2 sec off; repeat 5 times. Moving: In upright stance, move forwards and backwards and side to side, five steps each; repeat each movement 3 times.	Jab-cross combination (jab × 5 and cross × 5 for 5 rounds; 5 sec rests between rounds)	2-2-2-2 pattern: 2 forward shuffles, 2 backward shuffles, 2 left shuffles, 2 right shuffles (see round 6)	Jab-cross-duck: 2 forward shuffles, jab-cross-duck, 2 backward shuffles, jab-cross-duck, 2 left shuffles, jab-cross-duck, 2 right shuffles, jab-cross-duck
Cool-down	Hamstring and calf stretch (20-30 sec each leg); outward and inward shoulder stretch (20-30 sec each shoulder); and lying knee to chest (20 sec each leg)			

Intermediate 15-Minute Express Workout

The intermediate 15-minute express workout in figure 8.4 offers you the opportunity to take your skills to the next level by performing balance, coordination, strength and stamina exercises that are more challenging than those in the basic workout.

FIGURE 8.4   Intermediate 15-Minute Express Workout

Warm-up	Perform the basic warm-up, intermediate warm-up or advanced warm-up from round 5.			
Main session	Stance and guard: Upright stance and midlevel guard for 5 sec on, 2 sec off; repeat 5 times; maintain mid-level guard while moving forwards and backwards and side to side for 5 steps each; repeat each 3 times.	Jab-cross combination (jab-cross for 3 rounds at 60 sec each round; 15 sec rests between rounds)	2-2-2-2 pattern: 2 forward shuffles, 2 backward shuffles, 2 left shuffles, 2 right shuffles (3 rounds at 60 sec each round; 15 sec rests between rounds) (see round 6)	30-30 punch blast: (jab-cross combination for 30 sec with 30 sec rests between rounds; repeat for 3 rounds)
Cool-down	Hamstring and calf stretch (20-30 sec each leg); outward and inward shoulder stretch (20-30 sec each shoulder); and lying knee to chest (20 sec each leg)			

Advanced 15-Minute Express Workout

The advanced 15-minute express workout in figure 8.5 offers a fast-paced, high-energy workout that combines more complex and highly rewarding techniques, skills and drills that focus both the mind and body on each specific area to achieve maximum potential and amazing total-body results. Combining speed, power, strength and endurance along with the Total Knockout Fitness cutting-edge mind and body integration techniques, this advanced workout will leave you looking and feeling great.

FIGURE 8.5   Advanced 15-Minute Express Workout

Warm-up	Perform the basic warm-up, intermediate warm-up or advanced warm-up from round 5.			
Main session	Squat punch (3 rounds at 60 sec each round; 15-20 sec rests between rounds)	Twist jump and punch (3 rounds at 60 sec each round; 15 sec rests between rounds)	2-2-2-2 pattern: 2 forward shuffles, 2 backward shuffles, 2 left shuffles, 2 right shuffles (3 rounds at 60 sec each round; 15 sec rests between rounds) (see round 6)	Squat jump shuffle (3 rounds at 60 sec each round; 20 sec rests between rounds)
Cool-down	Hamstring and calf stretch (20-30 sec each leg); outward and inward shoulder stretch (20-30 sec each shoulder); and lying knee to chest (20 sec each leg)			

Now that you can combine footwork with punch combinations and have learned all the techniques you need to improve your performance, it is time to move on to the last part of this book: putting all your skills together. In the next rounds, you will learn about flexibility, weight loss, toning and shaping and more.

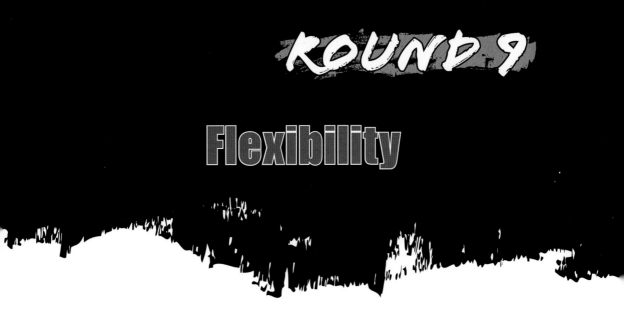

ROUND 9

Flexibility

You may have started the Total Knockout Fitness programme to get fitter, lose some weight or simply get in shape and tone your body. At this point you have probably started to see some results. However, to improve not just the way your body looks to yourself and others but also how you feel within, better flexibility can do wonders. A body that holds less tension and moves with less effort or pain will make you feel better from the inside out. This round is about improving your flexibility so you can exercise effectively and move with ease in every direction. With greater flexibility, you can increase your fitness level, burn more calories and shape up to achieve a real knockout physique. Let's start with a look at what flexibility is and the types of flexibility.

What Is Flexibility?

Your level of flexibility is determined by the range of movement (ROM) in one or more joints when performing a certain exercise, with or without equipment or a partner.

Your level of flexibility is influenced by a variety of internal factors such as the type of joint (e.g., in the shoulder, back or hip area); the joint's internal resistance to move; the bone structure surrounding the joint; the elasticity of the muscle tissue, tendons, ligaments or skin around the joint; and the temperature of the joint (joints are generally more flexible when they are warm). The external factors that affect your flexibility include the temperature of your training location (higher temperatures are generally linked to better flexibility), the time of day you are training (many people are more flexible in the afternoon than in the morning), your age (pre-adolescents tend to be more flexible than adults), your ability to perform a certain exercise and your commitment to achieving flexibility (the more you practise flexibility, the more flexible you will be).

Increasing your flexibility will help you achieve unrestricted and easy, smooth movements, which will make your workouts safer and more effective and everyday tasks easier. For example, an inflexible shoulder may make reaching up to a high cupboard difficult, and very tight leg muscles can strain your knees, making even everyday activities such as walking a strain. Reduced tension in your muscles is worthwhile because tight muscles perform less efficiently and may make you feel uncomfortable throughout your body.

The good news is that even if you are not very flexible at the moment, the Total Knockout Fitness programme will boost your flexibility with specific exercises and stretching routines. If you already have some degree of flexibility, you will find new ways to increase it even more, which will give you that extra boost to perform even better when working out. Following are a few ways to improve your flexibility.

Pay Attention to Your Shoulder Positions

Ideally, your shoulders should be pulled slightly back to avoid rounding them. Your muscles are designed to hold your body in correct alignment when they are working correctly together. Imagine a central pole in a tent with two ropes attached that extend to either side. Now imagine that one is pulled tighter than the other. It is clear that the other must be loosened to accommodate the tighter rope. A key problem area for many people is the shoulder and chest area, which contains vital organs including the lungs. Restrictions in this area increase tension throughout the body. By paying particular attention to your posture, the rest of your body has the best chance of functioning as it is designed to.

Drink More Water

Water, a crucial ingredient in everyone's diet, increases flexibility by contributing to total-body relaxation and increased mobility of the joints. To stay healthy, you need to replace the fluid you lose when you are active and sweat. The amount you should drink to avoid getting dehydrated will vary depending on a range of factors, including your size, the temperature or climate and how active you are. However, as a guide, experts recommend that you drink about 1.2 to 2 liters of fluid every day. This works out to be about six to eight 200-millilitre (6.8 oz) glasses.

Remember to Stretch

Stretching the shoulders, chest muscles, hips and legs by following the ultimate flexibility booster workout will increase your flexibility and help you move with more ease and energy. Being flexible in one joint does not necessarily mean that you are flexible in your entire body; a flexible upper body does not guarantee a flexible lower body. This is why stretching is so important: to get the whole body in a state of heightened flexibility and benefit from flexible joints all over your body, and feeling better and healthier.

Types of Flexibility

Flexibility is divided into dynamic, or kinetic, flexibility, which involves moving muscles to bring a limb through its whole range, and static flexibility, which involves no such movement. Static flexibility is divided into static-passive and static-active flexibility. Static-passive flexibility is the ability to attain and maintain an extended position using your body weight or a piece of equipment such as a chair. Static-active flexibility is the ability to stretch an antagonist muscle using only the tension in the agonist muscle. An example of static-active flexibility is holding one leg out in front of you as high as you can. When you do this, you are stretching the hamstring (in this case, the antagonist) while the quadriceps and hip flexors (in this, case the agonists) are actually holding the leg up.

Benefits of Flexibility

The next section addresses the benefits a high level of flexibility on your body and mind, from avoiding frictions in your muscles, joints and bones, releasing tension and enhancing posture to simply gaining an improved feeling of well-being all over.

Reduce Friction in Muscles, Joints, and Bones

One very important benefit of following a good flexibility routine is the enhanced production of glycosaminoglycans. This gel-like substance keeps muscle fibres from sticking together, thereby increasing pain-free range of movement. Glycosaminoglycan also helps repair tendons and joints and reduces the friction and inflammation that results from bone surfaces rubbing together as in various forms of arthritis.

Release Tension

Having flexible joints, especially in the neck and back area, will help you release tension and relax your body. As you may know, stress and physical tension are closely linked; for example, stress caused by work or other commitments can result in headaches or muscle tension. The good news is that stretching can ease tension; stretching overly tight neck muscles, for instance, can increase blood flow to and from the head. Making time for simple stretching exercises can enhance mobility and mental and physical harmony, reduce pain and increase your sense of well-being.

Feel Better

A healthy level of flexibility increases your overall sense of well-being as moving becomes easier and you are able to perform your exercise routines more smoothly. With greater flexibility, you can enjoy every movement rather than suffering pain or having to strain and force your body into uncomfortable positions—something you should avoid.

Improve Posture

With good flexibility, you can use your full range of motion and connect with your natural movements, which will improve your posture. In this way you can avoid a rounded back and keep your head and chin in their correct positions, boosting the way you look and feel.

Poor flexibility can lead to muscular imbalances, which can lead to bad posture and even poorer flexibility. Posture and flexibility go hand in hand. To get your posture and flexibility on a better track, avoid the following:

- ✔ Jutting your chin forwards—this puts pressure on your neck, shoulders and spine and causes unnecessary wear and tear on your joints, which may result in pain, tension and longer-term injuries.
- ✔ Arching your back—this can cause your body to compensate by adjusting other muscles, which can lead to injury and pain.
- ✔ Extending your abdomen as this puts unnecessary pressure on your spine and back.

Improve Body Alignment

A stretching routine can improve your body alignment by increasing the flexibility of your joints and muscles. This can result in naturally smooth movements performed with ease and energy. A better body alignment can boost your confidence by making you feel better and stronger.

Avoid Injury or Reinjury

Good flexibility can reduce the possibility of aggravating or reinjuring joints and muscles because your muscles will not be as tight. Muscles and joints that move smoothly function much better in the long term.

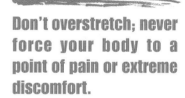

Don't overstretch; never force your body to a point of pain or extreme discomfort.

Total Knockout Fitness Ultimate Flexibility Booster Workout

Now it is time to step it up a notch and show you how an overall flexibility workout (see figure 9.1), from warm-up to cool-down, can not only boost your flexibility and improve your posture but also increase the toning and shaping of specific areas such as the arms, hips and legs.

FIGURE 9.1   Ultimate Flexibility Booster Workout

Warm-up	Perform the basic warm-up, intermediate warm-up or advanced warm-up from round 5.
Flexibility exercises	Perform 15 reps for each exercise: Hamstring and calf stretch Hip flexion with rotation Inward shoulder stretch Lunge with rotation Lying knee to chest Spiderman climb Total-body training stretch
Cool-down	Hamstring and calf stretch (20-30 sec each leg); outward and inward shoulder stretch (20-30 sec each shoulder); and lying knee to chest (20 sec each leg)

You now know more about how to increase your flexibility and hopefully have benefitted from the exercises and stretches in the ultimate flexibility booster workout by experiencing less tension and more flexibility in your joints and muscles. Releasing tension and increasing flexibility is a great way to improve your overall sense of well-being as you begin to move around with ease and perform everyday tasks and exercise routines more smoothly and safely. In the next few rounds you will learn how to improve your cardiorespiratory fitness, strength and power as well as super-effective ways to lose weight and get in great shape. So let's keep it moving: round 10 here we come!

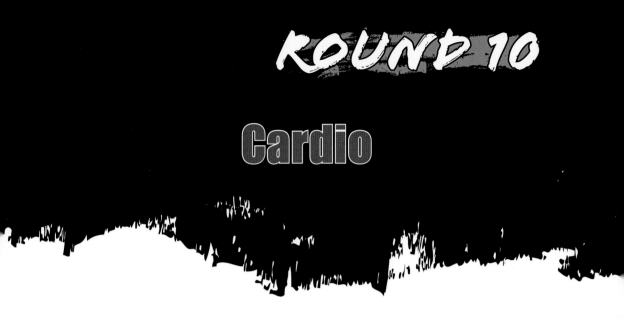

ROUND 10

Cardio

If you want to get in tiptop shape by burning calories at high speed with fun cardio-focused workouts, look no further. In this round you will learn how to boost your cardiorespiratory fitness by integrating fun exercises and boxing moves into your workout routine. This intense training programme will have you looking and feeling great and can be tailored to your current level of cardiorespiratory fitness. Get your body moving in all the right ways to burn calories at high speed and get in shape by following these new, total-body workouts.

In this round you will discover what cardiorespiratory fitness is, its benefits and how you can increase and maintain your level. You will learn how a balanced cardio workout programme can improve both your body and mind and how an efficiently working cardiovascular system can improve your health. This round can change your health and fitness enormously and gives you a great chance to establish some good fitness and health goals—both short and long term.

What Is Cardio?

Cardiorespiratory fitness (also called cardio, which we will use throughout this round) has to do with the ability of your heart, lungs and vascular system to take in, transport and use oxygen. *Cardio* refers to the heart, and *respiratory*, to the lungs. When referring to exercise, we use the term *cardiorespiratory*, although many use the term interchangeably with *cardiovascular*. *Vascular* refers to the network of arteries and veins that carry blood throughout the body. Regular, safe exercise improves the cardiovascular system by making the heart more efficient at pumping oxygen-rich blood, and the body more efficient at using oxygen. When you take a breath, oxygen goes straight into your bloodstream; your heart then pumps the oxygen-rich blood around your body, which energises your muscles.

Your cardiovascular system can be significantly compromised if you do not exercise regularly. With a higher level of cardiorespiratory fitness, your heart will do a better job of bringing oxygen to your muscles and all your body systems. This is why achieving and maintaining a high level of cardiorespiratory fitness is so crucial. You can incorporate the workout routines in this round into other routines or enjoy them as stand-alone routines focused on giving you that extra level of fitness.

Cardiorespiratory Fitness Factors

Improving your cardiorespiratory fitness is all about getting the intensity and duration of your workout right. The factors addressed in the following sections determine how successful you will be at boosting your cardio level.

Exercise Frequency

Although the American Heart Association recommends undertaking 30 minutes of activity at least five days of the week to keep your heart and lungs fit and strong, we recommend that you engage in moderate-to-vigorous exercise at least three times per week to boost your cardiorespiratory fitness. This round includes workouts that will make you work faster, harder and with super focus to achieve and maintain a cardio level that will keep you healthy and happy in body and mind.

Exercise Intensity

Exercise intensity refers to how hard your body is working; it varies from person to person. The level of intensity affects the fuel (i.e., carbohydrate or fat) your body uses and the adaptations of your body to the exercise (e.g., muscle growth and definition or body fat reduction). You can use a heart rate monitor during exercise to determine your intensity.

We recommend that you work at 70 to 85 percent of your maximum heart rate, which is calculated as 220 bpm (beats per minute) minus your age. If you are 35 years old, you would have a maximum heart rate of 185 bpm (220 − 35 = 185). Therefore, you would need to work out within a range of 129 to 157 bpm.

Exercise Duration

To take your cardiorespiratory fitness to the next level and maintain that level, you should exercise for 15 minutes to 1 hour per workout. For cardiorespiratory benefits you need to exercise for at least 12 minutes; this is a good starting point if you are new to exercise. As your workout sessions progress, gradually increase your duration. Cardiorespiratory, or aerobic, fitness refers to your ability to exercise for an extended period of time. This is also referred to as cardiorespiratory endurance. During aerobic activity, you use oxygen to break down fat and carbohydrate for energy.

Anaerobic exercise is working without the use of oxygen; this can be maintained only for short periods of time. The anaerobic energy system is used for short bursts of energy and intensity such as short sprints and anything that requires an intense burst of muscular activity. These powerful physical bursts of energy last, on average, 1 to 15 seconds. After that, you move back to aerobic activity, which means that you are again using oxygen.

Exercise Structure

Following a workout structure that involves your whole body and performing exercises, skills and drills to boost your cardiorespiratory fitness are essential for achieving your goals and maybe even exceeding your expectations. Having a clear plan or structure for your exercise routine (e.g., a specific time every week allocated to it) can help you stick to it. When you start to experience the positive changes to your body and energy levels, following your exercise structure becomes easier.

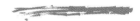

In the next part of this round you will get to know fun, calorie-busting punch drills that you can use as part of your cardio workout routine.

Benefits of Cardio Exercise

Enhancing your cardio level can be hugely beneficial to both body and mind, from improving your heart's efficiency and strength to reaching a healthy weight so you can feel and look better, fitter and healthier. The following sections outline the benefits of boosting your cardio level.

Improve Your Heart

When you exercise, your heart beats faster to meet your body's increased demand for oxygen. Your breathing and your body temperature increase, and at some point you may begin to sweat. All of these are indications that changes are taking place in your body. As you gradually stop exercising, your heart and breathing rate go back to normal and your body cools down.

50-Punch Countdown

This super-effective and intense boxing drill can be integrated into any workout to give you that cutting-edge cardio element. The 50-punch countdown will get you sweating and boost your cardio level in no time! Simply add it to the last part of your main session.

Using all of the techniques you've learned so far, here is the routine for the 50-punch countdown: jab-cross-jab-cross combination × 30 and then a left hook-right hook-left hook-right hook combination × 20. After each combination, make sure to move back to the Total Knockout Fitness upright stance and midlevel guard position.

This process has a very positive effect on your body and, in particular, your heart, especially once you start exercising regularly. The following sections outline the effects regular exercise and following a safe, structured cardio workout routine can have on your heart.

Lower Your Resting Heart Rate (RHR)

A heart that has the benefit of regular exercise actually beats fewer times at rest (resting heart rate, or RHR). Once you get into a regular exercise routine and become fitter, your resting heart rate decreases. As your fitness increases, the heart muscle gets stronger, pumping more blood through the heart with each beat, which means fewer beats per minute.

Reduce Your Recovery Time

A heart exposed to regular exercise takes less time to recover and return to its baseline after a workout. The fitter you become, the shorter your recovery time becomes. The time it takes your heart to return to its pre-exercise baseline is a measure of how fit you are: the shorter the recovery time, the fitter you are.

Boost Your Overall Health

With a stronger and more efficient heart, you are less at risk of a heart attack, stroke and diabetes. Exercising regularly can also decrease your bad cholesterol level, resulting in less plaque in your arteries so that your blood can flow more freely to and from your heart.

Lose or Maintain Weight

Not only can performing a structured cardio workout routine boost your cardiorespiratory fitness, but doing so can also help you lose or maintain weight. A little bit of cardio work can do a lot to bring you one step closer to your ideal weight. Keep in mind that weight loss is a focus for many people when they start an exercise routine, but cardio workouts provide many other health and fitness benefits as well.

Feel Better

Let's be honest, as much as working out sometimes seems to be 'too hard to bother', once you actually go for it and have a good workout, your body feels a great deal better. Right or wrong? So if you can feel energised and flexible after just one workout, imagine how great you will feel if you keep to an exercise routine of three times per week! Working out regularly not only boosts your energy and confidence levels, but also has amazing benefits for your mind, releasing stress and tension and leaving you feeling happier and more balanced. With a body that gets exercise frequently you will have more energy and less stress, and you will probably even sleep better.

Look Better

Cardio routines can greatly enhance your physical endurance. They allow you to burn through calories at high speed, shaping and toning areas you always wanted to improve.

Now that you know the benefits of achieving and maintaining a high level of cardiorespiratory fitness, you probably want to know how to improve your own level. The rest of this round outlines the ultimate cardio booster workout, which can bring amazing benefits to your health and the way you look and feel, and boost your confidence. All you need to invest is motivation and determination. This total-body workout will give your cardiorespiratory fitness a real boost, while burning fat and getting you in tiptop shape.

Total Knockout Fitness Ultimate Cardio Booster Workouts

The Total Knockout Fitness ultimate cardio booster workouts provide fun, simple ways of warming up, followed by intense, sweat-breaking main sessions and finishing off on a high with some stretching techniques to help you recover from your exercise session. So here we go—let's boost your cardio level once and for all!

If you are a beginner, it is best to start with the basic ultimate cardio booster workout and move to the intermediate workout after two weeks and then to the advanced workout. If you already have an established fitness routine, start with the intermediate and then move on to the advanced workout.

Basic Ultimate Cardio Booster Workout

The goal of the basic workout in figure 10.1 is to kick-start your cardiorespiratory fitness with an intense routine that will also tone your arms, glutes and legs. If you are new to exercise or have not exercised for a while, this workout is a great way to get you started on increasing your cardio level.

Intermediate Ultimate Cardio Booster Workout

The goal of the intermediate workout in figure 10.2 is to take your cardiorespiratory fitness to the next level by making your body work harder and thus burn more calories. If you have tried the basic cardio booster workout and feel that it does not challenge you enough, or if you already have a sound level of cardiorespiratory fitness, the intermediate cardio booster workout will be just right for you.

FIGURE 10.1 Basic Ultimate Cardio Booster Workout

Warm-up	Perform the basic warm-up, intermediate warm-up or advanced warm-up from round 5.		
Flexibility exercises	*Perform 2-3 exercises for 1 minute each:* Bend and flex, hamstring and calf stretch, hip flexion with rotation, hip rotation, inward shoulder stretch, lateral lunge, lunge with rotation, lying knee to chest, outward shoulder stretch, plank with rotational reach, single-leg wall reach, spiderman climb, toe reach and touch, or total-body training stretch		
Main session	Punch blast (2 rounds at 2 min each with 45 sec rests between rounds)	Footwork drill (2 rounds at 2 min each with 45 sec rests between rounds) (see round 6) Footwork clock drill Combination drill Shuffle punch footwork drill	PHA circuit: press-up; star jump; squat jump (20 sec each exercise for 2 full circuits with 2 min rests between circuits)
Cool-down	Hamstring and calf stretch (20-30 sec each leg); outward and inward shoulder stretch (20-30 sec each shoulder); and lying knee to chest (20 sec each leg)		

FIGURE 10.2 Intermediate Ultimate Cardio Booster Workout

Warm-up	Perform the basic warm-up, intermediate warm-up or advanced warm-up from round 5.		
Flexibility exercises	*Perform 2-3 exercises for 1 minute each:* Bend and flex, hamstring and calf stretch, hip flexion with rotation, hip rotation, inward shoulder stretch, lateral lunge, lunge with rotation, lying knee to chest, outward shoulder stretch, plank with rotational reach, single-leg wall reach, spiderman climb, toe reach and touch, or total-body training stretch		
Main session	Punch blast (2 rounds at 2 min each with 45 sec rests between rounds)	Footwork drill (2 rounds at 2 min each with 30 sec rests between rounds) Footwork clock drill Combination drill Shuffle punch footwork drill	PHA circuit: press-up; high-knee raise with lateral leap; star jump; bridge to plank; multidirectional squat thrust; squat (20 sec each exercise for 2 full circuits with 2 min rests between circuits)
Cool-down	Hamstring and calf stretch (20-30 sec each leg); outward and inward shoulder stretch (20-30 sec each shoulder); and lying knee to chest (20 sec each leg)		

Advanced Ultimate Cardio Booster Workout

The goal of the advanced workout in figure 10.3 is to super-boost your cardiorespiratory fitness. This workout, with its slightly more challenging drills, is for you if you already have a high level of cardiorespiratory fitness and want to take it one step further.

FIGURE 10.3   **Advanced Ultimate Cardio Booster Workout**

Warm-up	Perform the basic warm-up, intermediate warm-up or advanced warm-up from round 5.			
Flexibility exercises	*Perform 2-3 exercises for 1 minute each:* Bend and flex, hamstring and calf stretch, hip flexion with rotation, hip rotation, inward shoulder stretch, lateral lunge, lunge with rotation, lying knee to chest, outward shoulder stretch, plank with rotational reach, single-leg wall reach, spiderman climb, toe reach and touch, or total-body training stretch			
Main session	Punch blast (3 rounds at 2 min each with 45 sec rests between rounds)	Footwork drill (3 rounds at 2 min each with 30 sec rests between rounds) Footwork clock drill Combination drill Shuffle punch footwork drill	PHA circuit: press-up; high-knee raise with lateral leap; star jump; bridge to plank; multidirectional squat thrust; squat (30 sec each exercise for 3 full circuits with 2 min rests between circuits)	50-punch countdown (as described earlier in this round)
Cool-down	Hamstring and calf stretch (20-30 sec each leg); outward and inward shoulder stretch (20-30 sec each shoulder); and lying knee to chest (20 sec each leg)			

If you want to take your cardiorespiratory fitness even further, you can integrate other sport activities, such as running, into your cardio workout. For example, you can include an 800-metre interval in your workout routine regularly to give your cardio an extra boost.

Start with a three-minute warm-up combination of jogging, hopping and short sprints. Then move on to three 45-second to 1-minute intervals at medium intensity, with one- to two-minute rests between them. Follow this with three 25-second intervals at high intensity, interspersed with 30-second rests, and jog back to the starting point after each interval. End with a slow two-minute jog to cool down. For best results, perform two interval training sessions per week.

Phew! This round should have gotten you sweating. Now it is time to move on to the next part of this programme and discover how boxing for fitness can support and even accelerate weight loss in a healthy and balanced way. Round 11, here we come!

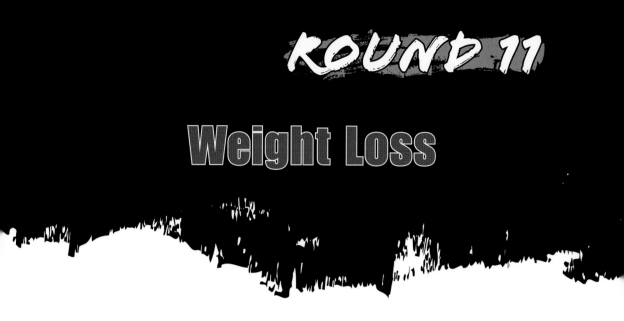

ROUND 11

Weight Loss

Round 11 offers unique insight into how to lose weight in a healthy way by following a simple, structured workout routine teamed up with a healthy, delicious diet that boosts your body with all the right nutrients to maximise fat and calorie burning while working out. It also addresses what to do before you even start your weight-loss programme, how to keep your motivation high throughout the programme, how to maximise your focus and determination and how to integrate healthy nutritional choices and a balanced exercise routine into your lifestyle.

What Is a Successful Weight-Loss Plan?

This round outlines a healthy, sensible approach to losing weight, not the miraculous, unrealistically fast and sometimes unhealthy or even dangerous approaches many people undertake. When you commit to following a holistic weight-loss plan that integrates a balanced exercise routine with a healthy diet over a specific period of time, you will start to see great results. The benefits of following this plan are positive health changes that will last so you can perform at your best.

Elements of Weight-Loss Success

You may have tried losing weight before and not succeeded in the way you would have liked. If this is the case, don't worry. You are not alone. Lots of people have tried to lose weight by following a specific programme or the latest diet craze and given up because they lost motivation or interest, could not keep up with the routine or simply did not see the desired results. Why do so many attempts at dropping weight end shortly after they start? The answer is that most people don't look at *all* the elements that a weight-loss programme should include. Many concentrate on only one aspect, such as giving up carbohydrate or eating more raw foods. Some try to lose weight by eating healthier and less food; others follow weight-loss programmes that overpromise and underdeliver. What can you do to succeed this time? The answer is to look at weight loss from a holistic point of view. If you integrate both a healthy diet and exercise into your lifestyle, you can achieve the weight you dream of.

In addition to diet and exercise, other elements factor into a successful weight-loss regime. The following sections offer tips to make sure your programme aids, rather than hinders, weight loss.

Set Realistic Goals and Expectations

Your body will take a while to adjust to the changes you make to your diet and will slowly get used to your exercise routine. Don't be disappointed if you don't lose an enormous amount of weight within the first days of changing your eating and exercise habits. It may take a while, but once your body is used to these positive changes, it will accept your new lifestyle and start working in your favour by burning fat more quickly, which will accelerate weight loss.

You may also find that the numbers on the scale are not shifting downwards as quickly as you hope, but that does not mean you have not made progress. Indicators other than your scale can reveal progress, such as the notches on your belt. Because muscle weighs more than fat, your weight may remain the same as your percentage of body fat decreases. Keep going and soon you will see real differences: on your body and on the scales.

Setting your weight-loss goal is the first step on your journey to losing weight healthily. To start, answer the questions in round 3 on setting your weight-loss goal and mini-goals. This can be a great motivator and keep you focused and engaged throughout the programme.

Avoid Distractions

The most important element of any weight-loss programme is staying focused, motivated and determined throughout. Whenever you don't feel motivated to get up and do your exercises, think about how you will look and feel once you lose that weight and are in better shape. Make sure you stick to a routine—that is, exercise on a specific day and at a specific time, when you will not be distracted by phone calls or friends or family coming in and out of the room. Keep distractions at bay by switching off your phone, TV and any of the other electronic devices that keep us entertained these days. Also, keep a clear space in which to work out, and plan enough time after the workout to relax a bit before getting started with the rest of your daily routine.

Fuel Your Body

To function at its best, your body must be fueled with the right foods. Round 3 gives you all the details on how to eat in a healthy and balanced way and how to boost your energy level while keeping within your optimum calorie intake. Whenever you need a bit of inspiration during your weight-loss journey, flip back to those pages that hold the key to a diet that is good for your body and your mind.

Lose Weight With the Right Exercise

To lose weight, you need to perform exercises that allow your body to burn calories much faster and to burn more fat. This will complement positive diet changes perfectly and accelerate weight loss. The exercises in this round are tailored to help you lose weight safely and healthily and in a balanced way, with tips and tricks for increasing your body's efficiency at burning calories. To lose weight and burn fat, you need to do the following:

- ✔ Set a time frame for your exercise programme that you can stick to (e.g., 12 weeks).
- ✔ Follow an exercise programme in which you expend more energy than you consume through your diet.
- ✔ Perform exercises that increase the amount of lean muscle tissue.
- ✔ Exercise often enough to increase your overall metabolism.
- ✔ Allow yourself time to rest. Don't exercise every day of the week; three or four times per week is plenty. If your body does not have enough time to recover from rigorous exercise, you may start feeling tired or even exhausted.

Weight-Loss Programme Benefits

Losing weight not only results in a leaner body but also improves your posture, boosts your confidence and increases your overall sense of well-being as a result of feeling fitter, healthier and more energetic. The following sections outline some of the benefits of losing weight.

Shape Your Body

The uniquely tailored weight-loss programme outlined in this round is designed to shape specific areas of your body. These exercises will tone your arms, bottom and legs while skyrocketing your fitness level and bringing you closer to your weight-loss goal.

Improve Your Posture

Following a high-quality weight-loss workout routine that tones and strengthens the muscles in and around your arms, shoulders and back will do wonders for your posture. This is one of the great benefits from the Total Knockout Fitness ultimate weight-loss programme.

Lose Weight

Of course, the most important benefit of a weight-loss programme is the weight loss itself. Keeping this in mind and picturing the way you will look and feel once you lose the desired amount of weight will help keep you on track and your motivation high.

Get Fit

Losing weight step by step using a balanced nutrition and exercise routine will make you fitter and healthier in many ways. You may experience increased energy, greater mental focus and concentration and improved range of mobility.

Prevent Disease

Losing weight has shown to be an effective tool in boosting overall health, by lowering blood pressure and reducing the risk of cardiovascular related disease. Sound nutrition and an effective exercise routine may even prevent type 2 diabetes. Such benefits may help you remain motivated to stay in shape over the long term.

Feel Better and More Confident

Losing weight will also increase your confidence as you watch your body change in shape and strength. The ultimate weight-loss workout outlined here will get you all the way to your desired weight-loss goal.

Total Knockout Fitness Ultimate Weight-Loss Workouts

The weight-loss workouts featured in this round, from basic to advanced, will put you on the right path for achieving your weight-loss goal. You will learn how to use specific exercises to accelerate your body's ability to lose weight in a balanced and healthy manner.

Basic Ultimate Weight-Loss Workout

The goal of the basic weight-loss workout in figure 11.1 is to kick-start your weight-loss programme. These fun exercises, including a warm-up and toning and shaping exercises, will accelerate the calorie- and fat-burning process. If you are new to exercise or have not exercised for a while but would like to take a first step in losing weight and reducing body fat, give the following workout a try.

FIGURE 11.1 **Basic Ultimate Weight-Loss Workout**

Warm-up	Perform the basic warm-up, intermediate warm-up or advanced warm-up from round 5.
Flexibility exercises	*Perform 2-3 exercises for 1 minute each:* Bend and flex, hamstring and calf stretch, hip flexion with rotation, hip rotation, inward shoulder stretch, lateral lunge, lunge with rotation, lying knee to chest, outward shoulder stretch, plank with rotational reach, single-leg wall reach, spiderman climb, toe reach and touch, or total-body training stretch

Main session	Shadowboxing: jab-cross (15 reps)	Squat jumps (15 reps each side)	Press-up (15 reps); side-to-side leaps (15 reps); bridge to plank (15 reps)	2-2-2-2 pattern (15 reps, 30 sec rests between sets) (see round 6)

Cool-down	Hamstring and calf stretch (20-30 sec each leg); outward and inward shoulder stretch (20-30 sec each shoulder); and lying knee to chest (20 sec each leg)

Intermediate Ultimate Weight-Loss Workout

The goal of the intermediate weight-loss workout in figure 11.2 is to take your regimen to the next level, adding intensity so that your body works slightly harder in all the right places to burn more fat. If you have been doing the basic weight-loss workout and seen some benefits but now feel as though you have reached a plateau, your body may need a bit more exercise. Time to try the intermediate workout!

Advanced Ultimate Weight-Loss Workout

The goal of this advanced weight-loss workout in figure 11.3 is to super-boost your weight loss so you can feel the amazing effects an intense weight-loss regimen can bring to your body and your mind. If you can easily manage the basic and intermediate weight-loss workouts outlined earlier and you would like to speed up your weight loss, try this advanced routine. These exercises will push you harder and speed up your body's ability to lose weight in all the right places.

FIGURE 11.2 Intermediate Ultimate Weight-Loss Workout

Warm-up	Perform the basic warm-up, intermediate warm-up or advanced warm-up from round 5.			
Flexibility exercises	*Perform 2-3 exercises for 1 minute each:* Bend and flex, hamstring and calf stretch, hip flexion with rotation, hip rotation, inward shoulder stretch, lateral lunge, lunge with rotation, lying knee to chest, outward shoulder stretch, plank with rotational reach, single-leg wall reach, spiderman climb, toe reach and touch, or total-body training stretch			
Main session	Shadowboxing: jab-cross (15 reps)	Squat (15 reps each side); press-up (15 reps); frontal leap (15 reps); bridge to plank (15 reps)	Speedball (up, down, forwards, backwards) for 5 reps each	Star jump (15 reps); bear crawl (15 reps)
Cool-down	Hamstring and calf stretch (20-30 sec each leg); outward and inward shoulder stretch (20-30 sec each shoulder); and lying knee to chest (20 sec each leg)			

FIGURE 11.3 Advanced Ultimate Weight-Loss Workout

Warm-up	Perform the basic warm-up, intermediate warm-up or advanced warm-up from round 5.			
Flexibility exercises	*Perform 2-3 exercises for 1 minute each:* Bend and flex, hamstring and calf stretch, hip flexion with rotation, hip rotation, inward shoulder stretch, lateral lunge, lunge with rotation, lying knee to chest, outward shoulder stretch, plank with rotational reach, single-leg wall reach, spiderman climb, toe reach and touch, or total-body training stretch			
Main session	Shadowboxing: jab-cross (15 reps)	Tuck jump (15 reps)	Star jump (15 reps); pendulum lunge (15 reps); bear crawl (15 reps); tuck jump (15 reps)	2-2-2-2 pattern (2 sets of 15 reps with 10 sec rests between sets) (see round 6)
Cool-down	Hamstring and calf stretch (20-30 sec each leg); outward and inward shoulder stretch (20-30 sec each shoulder); and lying knee to chest (20 sec each leg)			

Now that you are familiar with the holistic approach to weight loss, make sure you follow the recommended exercise schedule (three or four exercise sessions of up to 60 minutes per week, depending on your fitness level and how much weight you want to lose) and special diet recommended in round 3. Consider again how you can make healthy food choices to enhance your exercise routine and accelerate your weight loss. If you remain focused, determined and motivated, you will get your weight just where you want it to be. Fear the scales no more and stay on track with this programme to lose weight and you will feel great.

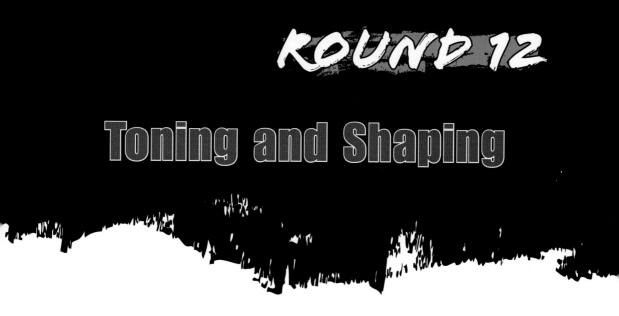

ROUND 12

Toning and Shaping

Getting toned and shaped with boxing and fitness workouts has never been easier! This round offers a range of tips and tricks for toning and shaping that body of yours in just the right areas with fun exercises and unique techniques. You will learn how toning and shaping exercises are performed and how to create a balanced, structured toning and shaping training programme that is based on fun cardio exercises and exciting boxing drills.

This round features a variety of total-body workout routines from a 15-minute express workout to three levels of ultimate toning and shaping workouts; these workouts will flatten your abdomen, lift your bottom and shape your waist, legs and arms, resulting in a real knockout physique. With routines tailored to various ability levels, you can choose the one that works best for you and progress safely to higher levels of challenge.

What Is Toning and Shaping?

People who want a more athletic physique that is not bulky or muscle bound often speak about toning and shaping the body. Muscles have a natural resting tone that can be increased by sticking to a regular exercise routine; shaping is achieved by increasing muscle tone while reducing body fat.

One of the main reasons many people start working out is to improve muscle definition and reshape their bodies. In general, exercises that promise to tone the body emphasise muscle building. The bad news is that no single exercise can tone all the muscles in your body; the good news is that a wealth of cardio exercises and boxing movements can reduce body fat, and body-weight exercises can build muscle definition. Performing a mix of such exercises and movements can result in 'toning', which translates as body leanness, low levels of body fat and noticeable muscle definition and shape. This condition promotes natural blood flow and an optimum range of movement, resulting in improved equilibrium and balance as well as a visually improved appearance.

To create a toned, shaped body, you must perform an exercise routine that creates healthy, oxygenated muscles that are the correct length for the bones they service. Muscle that is not toned contracts too much, which affects the performance of everyday activities or exercises. A muscle that is not the right length for the bone is either too tight or too lax. A muscle that is too tight can lead to constriction and unnecessary tension, and a muscle that is too lax can lead to hyperflexibility.

So how do you go about achieving leaner, healthier muscles? The following sections offer some tips to start your journey to a body with more defined muscles.

Set Toning and Shaping Goals

Setting goals is crucial for achieving the physique you want. Choose the number of workouts you want to do weekly, how and when you want to move from one level to another (i.e., upping the repetitions you are currently doing) and a specific time frame for getting in shape.

Push Hard

Working your body to its maximum will help enormously in toning and shaping your body. When performing these routines, stay focused, give them your all and don't give up. Staying on the ball and pushing your body will accelerate the process of creating the muscle definition you always wanted.

Mix It Up

Toning your body and losing weight will happen super-fast if you mix your toning exercises with effective cardio drills. The ultimate toning and shaping programme featured in this round provides a balance of cardio and toning exercises to help you meet your toning and shaping goals and lose weight throughout.

Follow a High-Rep Exercise Routine

Generally, low-rep, high-weight exercises increase strength and bulk. To achieve muscle definition, you need to perform more repetitions; this increases blood flow to your muscles, making them healthier and more defined while also burning fat. If you perform 20 reps per exercise and stick to it throughout your programme, you will start to see and feel results. The exercises in this round are a unique blend of boxing movements to boost muscle definition and cardio exercises to shape your body.

Mix Aerobic and Anaerobic Exercise

Mixing aerobic and anaerobic exercises will help you define muscle and burn fat—fast. Anaerobic exercises are exercises performed for short periods of time (up to 15 seconds) that don't use oxygen, such as explosive punch combinations or a fast punch countdown. Aerobic exercise is sustained for longer periods and uses oxygen; examples are a light jogging warm-up or punching or footwork drills done at a slower pace.

Include Retraction Exercises

Retraction exercises activate the back of your body and your postural muscles, resulting in a fitter-looking physique. Sitting at a desk in front of a computer for much of the day can have a negative effect on posture. If you feel your shoulders are rounding and you want to improve your posture, retraction exercises will help you stand straighter by strengthening your core muscles and lower back. Retraction exercises featured in the toning and shaping workouts are the dorsal raise and the advanced squat, in which you tense your fists and push your extended arms back as far as you can on the way back up, similar to an uphill skiing movement.

Eat and Drink to Accelerate Fat Burn

Foods and drinks that accelerate your body's fat-burning process include beetroot, apple cider vinegar, spicy foods and red peppers. And don't forget the all-important water!

Total Knockout Fitness Ultimate Shaping and Toning Workouts

As mentioned, you can improve your body shape and muscle definition by establishing and sticking to a regular, moderate-to-vigorous toning and shaping exercise regime. The following toning and shaping workouts include boxing and exercise techniques that will get your muscles working harder and faster to achieve the body shape you have always wanted.

Before getting into the specific workouts, you need to get the frequency and type of workouts right. For best results, choose your level of workout (basic, intermediate or advanced based on your level of fitness) and perform the corresponding workout schedule.

Basic

If you are just starting with exercise, this schedule will get you started slowly but steadily. Once you feel ready to move on (i.e., the exercises and reps are very manageable and you would like to challenge your body a bit more), move to the intermediate workout, which involves performing the routines more often.

✔ *2× per week*: basic ultimate toning and shaping workout (e.g., on Tuesday and Thursday)

✔ *3× per week*: 15-minute early riser express workout (e.g., on Monday, Wednesday and Friday)

Intermediate

If you are already used to exercising regularly (i.e., working out two or three times per week), following the intermediate workout schedule will take your exercise regimen to the next level and tone and shape your body more quickly.

✔ *3× per week*: intermediate ultimate toning and shaping workout

✔ *4× per week*: 15-minute early riser express workout

Advanced

If you are already exercising very regularly (e.g., three or four times per week) and you want to get super-toned and in even better shape, this workout schedule is for you.

✔ *4× per week*: advanced ultimate toning and shaping workout

✔ *5× per week*: 15-minute early riser express workout

15-Minute Early Riser Express Workout

This 15-minute workout (see figure 12.1) will kick-start your day and get you energised and super-focused while toning and shaping your body and oxygenating your system. Set your alarm clock 15 minutes earlier than usual and give this fun, short workout a go.

Total Knockout Fitness Ultimate Toning and Shaping Workouts

The ultimate toning and shaping programme in this section features superfast and ultra-effective toning and shaping workouts that include warm-ups, main sessions and cool-downs. Choose the one that suits your ability level and start getting in great shape while enjoying a holistic workout that will leave you feeling energised. These workouts target specific parts of your body, including your thighs, bottom, abdomen, chest and shoulders.

Basic Ultimate Toning and Shaping Workout

If you are new to exercise or have not exercised in a while, the basic workout routine in figure 12.2 will get you started on toning and shaping your body in a healthy and balanced way. This workout is perfect for kick-starting your healthy journey to a more shaped and toned physique.

FIGURE 12.1 15-Minute Early Riser Express Workout

Warm-up	Perform the basic warm-up, intermediate warm-up or advanced warm-up from round 5.		
Flexibility exercises	*Perform 2-3 exercises for 1 minute each:* Bend and flex, hamstring and calf stretch, hip flexion with rotation, hip rotation, inward shoulder stretch, lateral lunge, lunge with rotation, lying knee to chest, outward shoulder stretch, plank with rotational reach, single-leg wall reach, spiderman climb, toe reach and touch, or total-body training stretch		
Main session	Shadowboxing: straight cross 20× while focusing on a point	Two-speed press-up (20 reps)	Burpee (20 reps); dorsal raise (20 reps); ab crunch (20 reps); squat jump (20 reps)
Cool-down	Hamstring and calf stretch (20-30 sec each leg); outward and inward shoulder stretch (20-30 sec each shoulder); and lying knee to chest (20 sec each leg)		

FIGURE 12.2 Basic Ultimate Toning and Shaping Workout

Warm-up	Perform the basic warm-up, intermediate warm-up or advanced warm-up from round 5.				
Flexibility exercises	*Perform 2-3 exercises for 1 minute each:* Bend and flex, hamstring and calf stretch, hip flexion with rotation, hip rotation, inward shoulder stretch, lateral lunge, lunge with rotation, lying knee to chest, outward shoulder stretch, plank with rotational reach, single-leg wall reach, spiderman climb, toe reach and touch, or total-body training stretch				
Main session	Shadow-boxing: jab-cross (15 reps)	Jab (3 rounds of 10 punches with 15 sec rests between rounds)	Cross (3 rounds of 10 punches with 15 sec rests between rounds)	Jab-cross combination (3 rounds of 10 punches with 15 sec rests between rounds)	2-2-2-2 pattern: 3 rounds at 1 minute each with 20 seconds in between each round
Circuit session	Jump squat (30 sec); bridge to plank (30 sec); butt kickback (30 sec); triceps dip (30 sec); and plank (30 sec)				
Cool-down	Standing hamstring and calf stretch (30-40 sec each leg); standing quad stretch (30-40 sec each leg); lying knee to chest (30-40 sec each leg); upper-back reach stretch (30-40 sec); and static chest stretch (30-40 sec)				

Intermediate Ultimate Toning and Shaping Workout

If you are completely confident with and can easily perform the basic toning and shaping workout, you may want to challenge yourself some more by trying the intermediate workout in figure 12.3. It is a great way to further boost your toning and shaping experience and get results that you will see and feel. This workout is also perfect for you if you are already in good shape with a slightly toned body and want to get even more toned.

FIGURE 12.3 Intermediate Ultimate Toning and Shaping Workout

Warm-up	Perform the basic warm-up, intermediate warm-up or advanced warm-up from round 5.
Flexibility exercises	*Perform 2-3 exercises for 1 minute each:* Bend and flex, hamstring and calf stretch, hip flexion with rotation, hip rotation, inward shoulder stretch, lateral lunge, lunge with rotation, lying knee to chest, outward shoulder stretch, plank with rotational reach, single-leg wall reach, spiderman climb, toe reach and touch, or total-body training stretch

Main session	Shadow-boxing (jab-cross-jab-cross combination for 15 reps and jab-cross-hook-hook combination for 15 reps)	Jab-cross-jab-cross combination (3 rounds of 10 reps of the combination with 15 sec rests between rounds)	Jab-cross-hook-hook combination (3 rounds of 10 reps of the combination with 15 sec rests between rounds)	Jab-cross-duck combination (3 rounds of 10 reps of the combination with 15 sec rests between rounds)	2-2-2-2 pattern (3 rounds at 1 min each with 20 sec rests between rounds) (see round 6)

Circuit session	Squat jump (40 sec); press-up (40 sec); reverse lunge with rotation (40 sec); triceps dip (40 sec); and plank with alternate leg raise (40 sec)
Cool-down	Standing hamstring and calf stretch (30-40 sec each leg); standing quad stretch (30-40 sec each leg); lying knee to chest (30-40 sec each leg); upper-back reach stretch (30-40 sec); and static chest stretch (30-40 sec)

Advanced Ultimate Toning and Shaping Workout

If you are already toned or feel less than challenged by the basic and intermediate workout (or both), or if you want to add super-definition to your body, the advanced workout routine in figure 12.4 is for you. This routine will make a lasting difference to your body's tone and shape. If you stick to it, you will enjoy the results.

FIGURE 12.4   Advanced Ultimate Toning and Shaping Workout

Warm-up	Perform the basic warm-up, intermediate warm-up or advanced warm-up from round 5.				
Flexibility exercises	*Perform 2-3 exercises for 1 minute each:* Bend and flex, hamstring and calf stretch, hip flexion with rotation, hip rotation, inward shoulder stretch, lateral lunge, lunge with rotation, lying knee to chest, outward shoulder stretch, plank with rotational reach, single-leg wall reach, spiderman climb, toe reach and touch, or total-body training stretch				
Main session	Shadow-boxing (jab-cross-hook-hook combination for 15 reps and 2 upper-cuts-2 hooks for 15 reps)	Jab-cross-hook-hook combination (3 rounds of 10 reps of the combination with 15 sec rests between rounds)	Upper-cut-upper-cut-hook-hook combination (3 rounds of 10 reps of the combination with 15 sec rests between rounds)	Jab-cross-hook-hook-duck combination (3 rounds of 10 reps of the combination with 15 sec rests between rounds)	2-2-2-2 pattern (3 rounds at 1 min each with 20 sec rests between rounds) (see round 6)
Circuit session	Jumping squat (45 sec); press-up and hold (45 sec); reverse lunge with rotation (45 sec); triceps dip (45 sec); and plank with alternate leg raise (45 sec)				
Cool-down	Standing hamstring and calf stretch (30-40 sec each leg); standing quad stretch (30-40 sec each leg); lying knee to chest (30-40 sec each leg); upper-back reach stretch (30-40 sec); and static chest stretch (30-40 sec)				

You now know how to get your body toned and shaped by setting goals and staying with your workout routine. In round 13 you will learn some fun boxing workouts for building strength and power.

ROUND 13

Strength and Power

Some people are intimidated by the phrase *strength and power training;* they imagine men and women with bulging biceps and triceps and rippling abdominal muscles. Rest assured, this is not what this round is about. Round 13 focuses on increasing your fitness and health benefits by improving your strength and power through a variety of fun, explosive boxing moves and exhilarating exercises. The Total Knockout Fitness ultimate strength and power booster workouts are super-effective routines that can be tailored to your ability level so you can achieve the results you are looking for. The strength and power training routines featured in this round include body weight–based exercises and boxing moves that will enhance your strength without the need for any exercise or boxing equipment.

The good news is that strength and power can have a very positive influence on your overall boxing performance. Because they give your punches that extra power and allow you to punch with more impact, improving your strength and power is definitely worth your while.

What Is Strength and Power?

Strength can be defined as the extent to which your muscles can exert force by contracting against resistance (e.g., holding or restraining an object or person). Within this programme strength reflects your muscles' ability to produce force and power as well as to produce force at speed. This round will help you increase your power and strength by developing a base level of conditioning and then using explosive movements and exercises to gradually increase these two important elements of fitness and health.

Power is the ability to exert maximum muscle force in the shortest amount of time and is a combination of three factors—speed, strength and force. Training to increase power involves high-speed exercises executed with explosive movements to recruit as many muscles as possible. For example, when performing a jab-cross combination, you drive from the balls of the feet and up through the legs, rotating through the hips and torso with the shoulder following through before the arm extends the fist towards the target. You use both upper- and lower-body muscles to perform a smooth and swift boxing combination.

Ways to Improve Power and Strength

The Total Knockout Fitness programme focuses on increasing your muscles' strength and power gradually by integrating safe and fun body-weight exercises alongside explosive movements. This ensures that you benefit in your strength and power in all the right ways.

The following sections explain how body-weight exercises and explosive movement can make great changes to your strength and power.

Body-Weight Exercises

The training featured in this round includes body-weight exercises and boxing moves that will enhance your strength without the need for any exercise or boxing equipment. Using your own body weight to get stronger is not just good news for your wallet; it is also a highly effective way of toning and strengthening your body while simultaneously increasing your fitness level.

Body-weight exercises require you to support the weight of your body with one or more of your limbs, or to use your core muscles to lift your limbs against gravity's resistance. The frequent performance of body-weight exercises boosts muscular and cardiorespiratory fitness and improves psychomotor skills such as balance, agility and coordination. You can also increase your strength and mobility with movements such as bending, jumping, swinging, twisting and kicking using only your body weight for resistance.

Explosive Movement Exercises

Because boxing involves bursts of maximum speed and power, it is a great way to release feel-good endorphins as well as stress and tension—fast. You can achieve maximum speed by integrating explosive movements into your exercise regimen to develop strength and power. The boxing movements and exercises used in the routines in this round will help you generate maximum power because of their total-body action and high number of muscles recruited. Exercises that involve explosive movements are very intense and are done at full speed, which makes them an amazing tool for burning fat—fast. They also recruit more muscle fibres more frequently, which results in a leaner, more toned body.

Benefits of Strength and Power

Now that you understand the terms *strength* and *power*, let's have a look at the benefits you get from improving these two factors of your fitness.

Strengthen Your Muscles

By making your muscles stronger (using correct techniques), you will be more flexible and less prone to injuries. As you follow a strength regimen, not only do your muscles strengthen, but your tendons, ligaments and connective tissues also strengthen, which makes your body more efficient and more resilient.

Achieve a Toned Physique

Following a balanced strength and power training routine will result in your muscles feeling and looking stronger and more toned. This will bring you a step closer to a more toned, knockout physique.

Feel Better

In addition to increasing strength, speed and power, your strength and power routine will leave you healthier and feeling better. It boosts the immune system and increases vitality by releasing extra energy; keeping your body busy is good for your health.

Total Knockout Fitness Ultimate Strength and Power Booster Workouts

You may ask yourself how two elements of fitness—strength and power—can benefit from the very same workout. The answer is simple: both elements benefit because strength is one of the two components of power (the second is speed). When you improve your strength, you are building a foundation for enhanced power. Power cannot be developed without a strong foundation. You can compare this to the stability of a house: If the foundation is not strong enough, unforeseen circumstances could cause the house to crumble to pieces.

To see improvements of strength and power, we recommend that you train a minimum of three times per week, but no more than four to avoid the ill effects of overtraining. Because strength and power workouts are quite intense, your body needs to rest appropriately both after an exercise session and between reps and sets. If you are already working out more than four times per week, include a less intense workout session in your programme. Here is an example:

✔ *Monday, Tuesday and Thursday*—strength and power workout

✔ *Wednesday*—rest

✔ *Friday and Saturday*—flexibility workout

✔ *Sunday*—rest

This round features three levels of workout programmes. The basic workout is for those who are new to exercise or have not exercised for a while, and the intermediate is for those who want to take their strength and power to the next level. If you want to super-boost your strength and power with a more demanding routine, go for the advanced workout.

Basic Ultimate Strength and Power Booster Workout

If you are new to exercise or have not exercised for a while but want to work on your strength and power, this is the workout to opt for. This basic routine in figure 13.1 focuses on building your power and strength step by step; it includes exercises and boxing techniques that get your body slowly used to the demands of a power and strength workout.

FIGURE 13.1   **Basic Ultimate Strength and Power Booster Workout**

Warm-up	Perform the basic warm-up, intermediate warm-up or advanced warm-up from round 5.				
Flexibility exercises	*Perform 2-3 exercises for 1 minute each:* Bend and flex, hamstring and calf stretch, hip flexion with rotation, hip rotation, inward shoulder stretch, lateral lunge, lunge with rotation, lying knee to chest, outward shoulder stretch, plank with rotational reach, single-leg wall reach, spiderman climb, toe reach and touch, or total-body training stretch				
Main session	Four-punch power combo			Half burpee; press-up; squat jump; dorsal raise; plank (3 sets of 10-12 reps each exercise)	Low-intensity shadowboxing: Mix up and combining all techniques learned at a lower intensity (1 rep; 2 min rests between exercises).
	Jab-cross-jab-cross combination (5 reps with 1 min rests between reps)	Right hook-right hook-left hook-left hook combination (5 reps with 1 min rests between reps)	Right upper-cut-right upper-cut-left upper-cut-left uppercut combination (5 reps with 1 min rests between reps)		
Cool-down	Standing hamstring and calf stretch (30-40 sec each leg); standing quad stretch (30-40 sec each leg); lying knee to chest (30-40 sec each leg); upper-back reach stretch (30-40 sec); and static chest stretch (30-40 sec)				

Intermediate Ultimate Strength and Power Booster Workout

If you have already worked on your strength and power training elements and feel that the basic routine does not challenge you anymore, the intermediate workout routine in figure 13.2 is a great way to take your strength and power to the next level by increasing your reps in the main session.

FIGURE 13.2   **Intermediate Ultimate Strength and Power Booster Workout**

Warm-up	Perform the basic warm-up, intermediate warm-up or advanced warm-up from round 5.				
Flexibility exercises	*Perform 2-3 exercises for 1 minute each:* Bend and flex, hamstring and calf stretch, hip flexion with rotation, hip rotation, inward shoulder stretch, lateral lunge, lunge with rotation, lying knee to chest, outward shoulder stretch, plank with rotational reach, single-leg wall reach, spiderman climb, toe reach and touch, or total-body training stretch				
Main session	Four-punch power combo			Half burpee; press-up; squat jump; dorsal raise; plank (3 sets of 10-12 reps each exercise)	Low-intensity shadowboxing: Mix up and combine all techniques learned at a lower intensity (1 rep; 2 min rests between exercises).
	Jab-cross-jab-cross combination (8 reps with 1 min rests between reps)	Right hook-right hook-left hook-left hook combination (8 reps with 1 min rests between reps)	Right upper-cut-right upper-cut-left upper-cut-left uppercut combination (8 reps with 1 min rests between reps)		
Cool-down	Standing hamstring and calf stretch (30-40 sec each leg); standing quad stretch (30-40 sec each leg); lying knee to chest (30-40 sec each leg); upper-back reach stretch (30-40 sec); and static chest stretch (30-40 sec)				

Advanced Ultimate Strength and Power Booster Workout

If you are used to training strength and power and you want to super-boost these elements, then the advanced workout routine in figure 13.3 is for you. This workout integrates higher reps into your exercise routine, pushing your body just that bit harder to advance your strength and power to even higher levels.

FIGURE 13.3 **Advanced Ultimate Strength and Power Booster Workout**

Warm-up	Perform the basic warm-up, intermediate warm-up or advanced warm-up from round 5.					
Flexibility exercises	*Perform 2-3 exercises for 1 minute each:* Bend and flex, hamstring and calf stretch, hip flexion with rotation, hip rotation, inward shoulder stretch, lateral lunge, lunge with rotation, lying knee to chest, outward shoulder stretch, plank with rotational reach, single-leg wall reach, spiderman climb, toe reach and touch, or total-body training stretch					
Main session	Four-punch power combo			Footwork (forwards, backwards, left, right) for 1 min; shawdow-boxing with footwork (forwards, backwards, let, right) for 1 min	Half burpee; press-up; squat jump; dorsal raise; plank (4 sets of 10-12 reps each exercise)	Low-intensity shadow-boxing: Mix up and combine all techniques learned at a lower intensity (1 rep and 2 min rests between exercises).
	Jab-cross-jab-cross combination (10 reps with 1 min rests between reps)	Right hook-right hook-left hook-left hook combination (8 reps with 1 min rests between reps)	Right upper-cut-right upper-cut-left upper-cut-left uppercut combination (8 reps with 1 min rests between reps)			
Cool-down	Standing hamstring and calf stretch (30-40 sec each leg); standing quad stretch (30-40 sec each leg); lying knee to chest (30-40 sec each leg); upper-back reach stretch (30-40 sec); and static chest stretch (30-40 sec)					

Six Minutes to Strength and Power

If you want to work on your strength and power but don't have a lot of time to work out, this six-minute routine is a great alternative to the ultimate strength and power routines. You can do this as a stand-alone workout if you have only the six minutes it requires, or you can add it to any of the workouts featured in this book to add a strength and power training element. Here it is:

> One minute of skipping (to increase leg strength)

> Two minutes of a 20-punch countdown (alternate jab-cross-jab-cross until you reach 20 to enhance arm speed)

> Three minutes of squat jumps and burpees (alternate squats and burpees until you reach the end of the three minutes to improve power)

In this round you learned fun exercises for increasing your strength and power in a healthy and balanced way. Now it is time to take it the ultimate level. Let's go the extra (final) round!

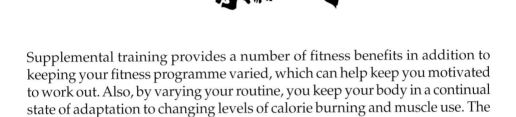

ROUND 14

Going the Extra Round

Supplemental training provides a number of fitness benefits in addition to keeping your fitness programme varied, which can help keep you motivated to work out. Also, by varying your routine, you keep your body in a continual state of adaptation to changing levels of calorie burning and muscle use. The supplemental training options featured in this round are fun alternatives to standard gym routines that provide both variety and holistic benefits.

The training choices in this round involve running, swimming and cycling. When integrated into a balanced Total Knockout Fitness workout routine, they add significant fitness and health benefits while enhancing your boxing performance by adding strength, speed and power to your upper and lower body.

Total Knockout Fitness Swimming Fusion

Swimming is a great add-on to your boxing workout routine because it boosts strength throughout your body. This will enhance your power when you execute punches and punch combinations and increase your overall cardiorespiratory fitness, which will come in handy when you perform head-turning footwork and skipping techniques.

Swimming is fun and burns lots of calories, is easy on your joints because the water supports your body weight, enhances muscular strength and endurance and improves your cardiorespiratory fitness level. The following list of benefits may be enough to inspire you to start swimming or take your swimming skills to the next level:

✔ *Is low impact*—Because it involves no ground impact, swimming is easy on your joints.

✔ *Develops cardiorespiratory fitness*—Swimming movements work your whole body thereby improving your endurance and increasing your oxygen consumption as well as strengthening your heart by enhancing stroke volume.

✔ *Enhances muscle mass*—Because you use your arms to glide your body forwards, swimming strengthens the triceps, enhancing your muscle tone.

✔ *Burns calories fast*—Swimming is an amazing calorie burner because of its naturally high level of intensity. Depending on the technique you are using and how efficiently you swim, you can burn 500 to 600 calories per hour, while enjoying benefits to your overall well-being.

Next we explore swimming techniques and how you can integrate a fun swimming routine into your Total Knockout Fitness programme to achieve an effective, total-body workout that is balanced and structured.

Swimming Styles

The Total Knockout Fitness programme uses the crawl, the backstroke and the breaststroke to create a balanced workout that fuses smoothly with the boxing skills you have already acquired.

Crawl

The crawl is a very popular stroke and the easiest for beginners to learn. It involves a simple flutter kick and windmill arm motion, just like the backstroke, only you are on your belly. The legs alternate in a flutter kick, with the knees bent slightly and the feet relaxed so they seem almost floppy. The down kick is emphasised for propulsion. At the same time, the arms move in an alternating windmill motion. Pulling both arms through the water with equal strength and reach will ensure that you swim straight. Underwater, the arms create an S pattern and the hands are cupped; the wrists and hands are relaxed during recovery.

Because your face is in the water most of the time during the crawl, you need to coordinate your breathing. When you raise one arm to begin the stroke your shoulder rises and you can lift your head just enough out of the water to take a quick breath. Take as many breaths as necessary and then exhale through your nose and mouth when your head returns to the water. Repeat the head turn to the other side in coordination with the beginning of the opposite arm stroke.

Breaststroke

The basics of the breaststroke are: arm pull, breath, kick (arms alternate with the kick), causing you to glide in a bob-up-and-down movement. The knees are brought to the chest and then the legs are thrust out and back until they are straight. The legs are then snapped together to push the water and propel you forwards (similar to a frog kick). The arms start overhead, and then pull on the water as they move towards the chest with hands cupped and performing a circular motion before returning to the starting position. You breathe every time you stroke with your arms.

Backstroke

The backstroke is similar to the crawl in that it involves an alternate wind-mill arm stroke and flutter kick. Move your arms with equal strength to avoid swimming off to one side, and roll your body from side to side so that your arms catch enough water to propel you forwards. The legs move in an alternating flutter kick, with the knees bent slightly and the feet relaxed so they seem almost floppy. The up kick is emphasised for propulsion. Bend the knees slightly.

During the backstroke the arms move in an alternating windmill pattern as they rotate and pass your face. The hands are cupped, and the thumb leaves the water first. The hands move in an S pattern when they are pushing the water. Keep your head back and eyes towards the ceiling. You can establish your own breathing pattern with the backstroke because your head should always be out of the water; you don't have to coordinate your breathing with your arm and leg movements as in other strokes.

Total Knockout Fitness Swimming Fusion Workouts

This section provides three levels of swimming fusion workouts. As mentioned, swimming offers great fitness benefits and is very low impact because the body is supported by the water. It is a great activity if you suffer from joint or muscular injuries or need to rehabilitate or strengthen your back. However, it is important to seek the advice of a medical professional before you commence any fitness programme, especially rehabilitation. By adding one or two swimming sessions a week to your normal fitness programme, you will soon experience the benefits. Swimming it is also a great way to involve family and friends in your fitness regimen.

Basic Swimming Fusion Workout

If you can swim safely but don't know the specific strokes, the basic workout in figure 14.1 is right for you. The goal this workout is to build your confidence with all of the swimming techniques through practice.

FIGURE 14.1   Basic Swimming Fusion Workout

Warm-up	Perform the basic warm-up, intermediate warm-up or advanced warm-up from round 5.		
Flexibility exercises	*Perform 2-3 exercises for 1 minute each:* Bend and flex, hamstring and calf stretch, hip flexion with rotation, hip rotation, inward shoulder stretch, lateral lunge, lunge with rotation, lying knee to chest, outward shoulder stretch, plank with rotational reach, single-leg wall reach, spiderman climb, toe reach and touch, or total-body training stretch		
Main session	Jab and cross (5 sets of 10 jabs with 8-10 sec rests between sets; 5 sets of 10 crosses with 8-10 sec rests between sets)	Jab-cross combination (5 sets with 8-10 sec rests between sets)	2-2-2-2-pattern: 2 forward shuffles, 1 jab-cross, 2 backward shuffles, 1 jab-cross, 2 left shuffles, 1 jab-cross, 2 right shuffles, 1 jab-cross (three 2 min rounds with 45 sec rests between rounds) (see round 6)
Basic swimming routine (30 min)	Choose a stroke you are comfortable with. As you feel ready, swim for five minutes without stopping and then take a break just long enough to catch your breath. Swim again for another five minutes, rest and then go again. After each break, change your swimming technique.		
Cool-down	Standing hamstring and calf stretch (30-40 sec each leg); walking quad stretch (30-40 sec each leg); lying knee to chest (30-40 sec each leg); and upper-back reach stretch (30-40 sec)		

Intermediate Swimming Fusion Workout

If you are confident in swimming for the 30 minutes required in the basic workout and you want a more challenging, more intense fusion workout, the intermediate workout in figure 14.2 is absolutely right for you. This workout will further strengthen your muscles and increase your endurance.

FIGURE 14.2 **Intermediate Swimming Fusion Workout**

Warm-up	Perform the basic warm-up, intermediate warm-up or advanced warm-up from round 5.		
Flexibility exercises	*Perform 2-3 exercises for 1 minute each:* Bend and flex, hamstring and calf stretch, hip flexion with rotation, hip rotation, inward shoulder stretch, lateral lunge, lunge with rotation, lying knee to chest, outward shoulder stretch, plank with rotational reach, single-leg wall reach, spiderman climb, toe reach and touch, or total-body training stretch		
Main session	Jab and cross (5 sets of 10 jabs with 8-10 sec rests between sets; 5 sets of 10 crosses with 8-10 sec rests between sets)	Jab-cross combination (5 sets with 8-10 sec rests between sets)	2-2-2-2 pattern: 2 forward shuffles, 1 jab-cross, 2 backward shuffles, 1 jab-cross, 2 left shuffles, 1 jab-cross, 2 right shuffles, 1 jab-cross (three 2 min rounds with 45 sec rests between rounds) (see round 6)
Intermediate swimming routine (30 min)	The intermediate swimming routine is all about varying your stroke styles and speed to further boost your fitness and burn even more calories. As you feel ready, swim 10 minutes performing a breaststroke, and then take a break long enough to catch your breath. Get right back to it and swim again for 5 minutes of the crawl, take a break and swim 10 minutes of the backstroke. Continue this pattern for a minimum of 30 minutes.		
Cool-down	Standing hamstring and calf stretch (30-40 sec each leg); walking quad stretch (30-40 sec each leg); lying knee to chest (30-40 sec each leg); and upper-back reach stretch (30-40 sec)		

Advanced Swimming Fusion Workout

If you have mastered all of the exercises and swimming routines prescribed in the basic and intermediate workouts and you want to boost your endurance, strength and cardio levels, you are ready for the advanced workout in figure 14.3.

FIGURE 14.3	Advanced Swimming Fusion Workout		
Warm-up	Perform the basic warm-up, intermediate warm-up or advanced warm-up from round 5.		
Flexibility exercises	*Perform 2-3 exercises for 1 minute each:* Bend and flex, hamstring and calf stretch, hip flexion with rotation, hip rotation, inward shoulder stretch, lateral lunge, lunge with rotation, lying knee to chest, outward shoulder stretch, plank with rotational reach, single-leg wall reach, spiderman climb, toe reach and touch, or total-body training stretch		
Main session	Jab and cross (5 sets of 10 jabs with 8-10 sec rests between sets; 5 sets of 10 crosses with 8-10 sec rests between sets)	Jab-cross combination (5 sets with 8-10 sec rests between sets)	2-2-2-2 pattern: 2 forward shuffles, 1 jab-cross, 2 backward shuffles, 1 jab-cross, 2 left shuffles, 1 jab-cross, 2 right shuffles, 1 jab-cross (three 2 min rounds with 45 sec rests between rounds) (see round 6)
Advanced swimming routine (30 min)	The focus of this swimming and boxing fusion workout (along with increasing your strength and endurance) is to boost your cardiorespiratory fitness level and create an exercise regimen that will increase your overall well-being and refresh your energy level. Starting at the edge of the pool, lower your body beneath the surface and push off with your legs; glide with your arms outstretched like a torpedo. As you begin to slow down, thrust your arms to your sides to provide a final boost and notice how far you have travelled. When you are ready, repeat this exercise for 3 minutes with the aim of furthering your distance each time. After 3 minutes, follow up with 5 minutes of the crawl, and then take a break long enough to catch your breath. Then, perform 10 minutes of the breaststroke, followed by 10 minutes of the backstroke and, finally, 2 minutes of the torpedo.		
Cool-down	Standing hamstring and calf stretch (30-40 sec each leg); walking quad stretch (30-40 sec each leg); lying knee to chest (30-40 sec each leg); and upper-back reach stretch (30-40 sec)		

Total Knockout Fitness Cycling Fusion

Cycling is a low-impact exercise with the great advantage of being easier on your joints than running or other high-impact aerobic activities, while still helping you to get in shape. It strengthens and shapes the whole body, especially the lower body (riding uphill works the upper body). Supplementing your training with regular cycling can accelerate weight loss, reduce stress levels and improve overall fitness. Following are other benefits:

✔ *Saves money and is kind to nature*—Cycling not only increases fitness but is also a form of transport, saving you money and making a positive contribution to the environment.

✔ *Burns calories*—Riding a bike works your whole body and helps you burn lots of calories. For example, if you weigh 80 kilograms (12 st or 9 lb), you will burn more than 600 calories in an hour of riding, and tone your legs and bottom in the process.

✔ *Improves your boxing performance*—Cycling increases the strength in your legs, which will benefit your footwork skills and increase your cardiorespiratory fitness. Following a balanced cycling routine will help you perform longer, faster boxing workouts because your endurance will be greater.

Cycling Safety

Cycling is a great, safe way to increase balance, timing and coordination along with strength and cardiorespiratory fitness. You can choose an intensity level to suit your preference, from a leisurely cycle with others to a more intense sprint or off-road ride. There really is something for everyone. Whether you try an exercise bike in the gym or at home or enjoy a ride to work or around the park, by adding one or two sessions a week to your training programme, you will see results.

When riding your bike, make sure you are wearing a cycling helmet to prevent a head injury in case of a fall. Make sure your helmet is snug and comfortable and sits above your eyebrows instead of being tilted backwards or forwards. Leave room for two fingers between your chin and the strap.

When out on the road, follow these safety tips:

✔ Always look behind you before you turn, overtake or stop.

✔ Use arm signals before you turn right or left. Before turning left, stretch your left arm out to the left side so people in cars, pedestrians, motorcyclists or other cyclists know that you are about to turn. When you want to turn right, stretch your right arm to the right side.

✔ Don't ride on the pavement (also called the sidewalk) unless a sign is posted saying you can.

✔ On busy or narrow roads, don't cycle next to another person.

✔ Obey traffic lights and road signs at all times.

✔ When overtaking parked cars, watch out for car doors opening suddenly and allow room to pass safely.

✔ Don't use headphones or mobile phones while cycling.

✔ Check that the lights on your bike are working (white front light, red rear light, red rear reflector and yellow or amber pedal reflectors on the front and back of each pedal).

Total Knockout Fitness Cycling Fusion Workouts

Adding a cycling fusion workout to your normal exercise regimen will result in noticeable changes to your cardiorespiratory fitness as well as your endurance and strength, especially in the thighs. This round offers three levels of cycling fusion workouts. Simply add the level of cycling workout you choose to your regular exercise routine. In addition to benefitting your fitness and health, cycling is also a great way to clear your mind and increase your energy level.

Basic Cycling Fusion Workout

The cycling fusion programme is a fun mix of boxing skills and cycling that will increase your overall cardiorespiratory fitness, balance and coordination. The basic workout in figure 14.4 integrates a light cycling routine into your training. If you live no farther than 20 minutes from your workplace, why not skip the car or public transport and ride to work? It's a great way to kick-start your day while increasing your fitness level. When you have mastered the basic workout and want to challenge yourself a bit more, move on to the intermediate workout.

FIGURE 14.4 Basic Cycling Fusion Workout

Warm-up	Perform the basic warm-up, intermediate warm-up or advanced warm-up from round 5.		
Flexibility exercises	*Perform 2-3 exercises for 1 minute each:* Bend and flex, hamstring and calf stretch, hip flexion with rotation, hip rotation, inward shoulder stretch, lateral lunge, lunge with rotation, lying knee to chest, outward shoulder stretch, plank with rotational reach, single-leg wall reach, spiderman climb, toe reach and touch, or total-body training stretch		
Main session	Jab and cross (5 sets of 10 jabs with 8-10 sec rests between sets; 5 sets of 10 crosses with 8-10 sec rests between sets)	Jab-cross combination (5 sets with an 8-10 sec rest between sets)	2-2-2-2 pattern: 2 forward shuffles, 1 jab-cross, 2 backward shuffles, 1 jab-cross, 2 left shuffles, 1 jab-cross, 2 right shuffles, 1 jab-cross (three 2 min rounds with 45 sec rests between rounds) (see round 6)
Basic cycling routine (30 min)	Choose a cycling route on relatively flat and smooth terrain that will take at least 30 minutes to complete at a steady, comfortable pace. This is a simple way to get you started before moving to the next level. If you can, chose a scenic route (e.g., through a park or on a nature trail) to make your ride more enjoyable.		
Cool-down	Standing hamstring and calf stretch (30-40 sec each leg); walking quad stretch (30-40 sec each leg); lying knee to chest (30-40 sec each leg); and upper-back reach stretch (30-40 sec)		

Intermediate Cycling Fusion Workout

The intermediate cycling fusion workout in figure 14.5 will boost your cardio level and strengthen the muscles in your lower body by having you perform different positions on your bike. When this routines starts to feel too easy, it is time to move to the advanced workout and provide your body with more vigorous, challenging exercises.

FIGURE 14.5   Intermediate Cycling Fusion Workout

Warm-up	Perform the basic warm-up, intermediate warm-up or advanced warm-up from round 5.		
Flexibility exercises	*Perform 2-3 exercises for 1 minute each:* Bend and flex, hamstring and calf stretch, hip flexion with rotation, hip rotation, inward shoulder stretch, lateral lunge, lunge with rotation, lying knee to chest, outward shoulder stretch, plank with rotational reach, single-leg wall reach, spiderman climb, toe reach and touch, or total-body training stretch		
Main session	Jab and cross (5 sets of 10 jabs with 8-10 sec rests between sets; 5 sets of 10 crosses with 8-10 sec rests between sets)	Jab-cross combination (5 sets with 8-10 sec rests between sets)	2-2-2-2 pattern: 2 forward shuffles, 1 jab-cross, 2 backward shuffles, 1 jab-cross, 2 left shuffles, 1 jab-cross, 2 right shuffles, 1 jab-cross (three 2 min rounds with 45 sec rests between rounds) (see round 6)
Intermediate cycling routine (30 min)	This more advanced routine works your thighs, increases your endurance and boosts your cardiorespiratory fitness even more. It can be performed on either a stationary or road bike. *0-5 minutes:* Cycle at a steady pace. *5-20 minutes:* Every minute and a half, include a 45-second stand-up in which you focus on your legs, bum and core muscles. *20-25 minutes:* Cycle up a hill as quickly as possible, return to the bottom and repeat. *25-30 minutes:* Cycle at a steady pace to cool down.		
Cool-down	Standing hamstring and calf stretch (30-40 sec each leg); walking quad stretch (30-40 sec each leg); lying knee to chest (30-40 sec each leg); and upper-back reach stretch (30-40 sec)		

Advanced Cycling Fusion Workout

The advanced cycling fusion workout in figure 14.6 combines the ultimate boxing for fitness skills with a fun stamina- and strength-boosting cycling workout so you can super-boost your overall health and fitness levels while getting in great shape.

FIGURE 14.6	Advanced Cycling Fusion Workout		
Warm-up	Perform the basic warm-up, intermediate warm-up or advanced warm-up from round 5.		
Flexibility exercises	*Perform 2-3 exercises for 1 minute each:* Bend and flex, hamstring and calf stretch, hip flexion with rotation, hip rotation, inward shoulder stretch, lateral lunge, lunge with rotation, lying knee to chest, outward shoulder stretch, plank with rotational reach, single-leg wall reach, spiderman climb, toe reach and touch, or total-body training stretch		
Main session	Jab and cross (5 sets of 10 jabs with 8-10 sec rests between sets; 5 sets of 10 crosses with 8-10 sec rests between sets)	Jab-cross combination (5 sets with 8-10 sec rests between sets)	2-2-2-2 pattern: 2 forward shuffles, 1 jab-cross, 2 backward shuffles, 1 jab-cross, 2 left shuffles, 1 jab-cross, 2 right shuffles, 1 jab-cross (three 2 min rounds with 45 sec rests between rounds) (see round 6)
Advanced cycling routine (30 min)	This routine focuses on increasing your stamina and further challenging your body with advanced cycling to super-boost your fitness level. It can be performed on either a stationary or road bike. *0-5 minutes:* Cycle at a steady pace. *5-17 minutes:* Every minute, include a two-minute stand-up in which you focus on your legs, bum and core muscles. *17-25 minutes:* Change resistance by using hills or gears, as available. *25-30 minutes:* Cycle at a steady pace to cool down.		
Cool-down	Standing hamstring and calf stretch (30-40 sec each leg); walking quad stretch (30-40 sec each leg); lying knee to chest (30-40 sec each leg); and upper-back reach stretch (30-40 sec)		

Total Knockout Fitness Running Fusion

Because running naturally boosts your cardiorespiratory fitness and endurance levels and your overall health, it is great supplemental training to add to your boxing workout routine. It will help you punch faster and last longer when performing footwork and skipping skills and drills.

According to the American College of Sports Medicine, Americans who ran more than 50 miles per week had significantly higher levels of HDL cholesterol (the good cholesterol) and significantly less body fat and risk of coronary heart disease than people who ran less than 10 miles per week. In addition, the long-distance runners had nearly 50 percent lower blood pressure and more than a 50 percent reduction in the use of medications to lower blood pressure and plasma cholesterol levels. Using running as part of your Total Knockout Fitness programme offers many benefits to your body and mind, including the following:

- ✔ *Improves cardiorespiratory fitness*—Running strengthens your heart so it can pump more blood with each beat and deliver more oxygen to your muscles. It increases your cardiorespiratory fitness by increasing the activity of enzymes and hormones that stimulate the muscles and the heart to work more efficiently.

- ✔ *Results in a more-defined and leaner physique*—Running is great for defining muscles, especially in the legs and arms because these are used at maximum capacity when running correctly.

- ✔ *Burns calories*—As a cardiorespiratory-based fitness activity, running is great for burning calories because it works your body hard and intensely.

- ✔ *Is easily adapted to any fitness level*—Running is a simple activity that can be adapted to your current fitness level and progressed as you become fitter. You can start with a brisk walk and gradually progress to a walk–run combination and finally to a continuous run.

- ✔ *Releases stress*—Running offers a great opportunity to de-stress, clear your mind and reenergise your body.

To gain maximum health and fitness benefits, integrate a running routine into your exercise session three to five days per week at 55 to 90 percent of your maximum heart rate. To get the heart, muscles and calorie-burning process working maximally, aim for 30 minutes of running per routine.

Proper Running Technique

As in any sport, technique is very important in running. Paying attention to your form will help you avoid injury and gain maximum benefits.

To run properly, keep your body erect and look forwards to the horizon with your chest lifted and out so you can breathe deeply and exhale fully. Your shoulders, face, jaw and torso should be relaxed to avoid unnecessary tension that can restrict your movement and breathing. Keep your arms close to your body and swing them forwards and backwards, not across your body, to minimise torso rotation. Your elbows should be relaxed at a 90-degree angle, and your hands should be cupped by gently touching your thumbs to the top half of your index fingers.

Total Knockout Fitness Running Fusion Workouts

This section provides three levels of running fusion workouts. Running offers many benefits, from the obvious cardiorespiratory and muscular benefits to stress busting and tension release. Many runners experience what they call the runner's high as a result of the feel-good hormones that running releases. As with cycling, you can choose the level you prefer, from a gentle jog to a sprint, and run either outside or on an indoor track or a treadmill in the gym or at home.

Begin running at an intensity level that is challenging but achievable and build from there. The benefits will depend on how often you run, but with each session you will start to notice an increase in your overall well-being. One or two sessions of moderate-intensity running per week is a good supplement to your Total Knockout Fitness programme.

Basic Running Fusion Workout

If you are just starting with running, the basic programme in figure 14.7 will get your body used to running at a steady pace as you slowly build your endurance. When the basic workout starts to feel too easy and you feel the need for more of a challenge, move on to the intermediate workout.

FIGURE 14.7   Basic Running Fusion Workout

Warm-up	Perform the basic warm-up, intermediate warm-up or advanced warm-up from round 5.
Flexibility exercises	*Perform 2-3 exercises for 1 minute each:* Bend and flex, hamstring and calf stretch, hip flexion with rotation, hip rotation, inward shoulder stretch, lateral lunge, lunge with rotation, lying knee to chest, outward shoulder stretch, plank with rotational reach, single-leg wall reach, spiderman climb, toe reach and touch, or total-body training stretch

Main session	Jab and cross (5 sets of 10 jabs with 8-10 sec rests between sets; 5 sets of 10 crosses with 8-10 sec rests between sets)	Jab-cross combination (5 sets with 8-10 sec rests between sets)	2-2-2-2 pattern: 2 forward shuffles, 1 jab-cross, 2 backward shuffles, 1 jab-cross, 2 left shuffles, 1 jab-cross, 2 right shuffles, 1 jab-cross (three 2 min rounds with 45 sec rests between rounds) (see round 6)

Basic running routine (30 min)	Aim for 30 minutes of activity that suits you but also challenges your current fitness level. Start with a five-minute brisk power walk to warm up. When you feel ready, start to jog. If you get out of breath, slow down and keep jogging or power walk again until you catch your breath. This could take one to two minutes. Aim to reduce the time you are power walking as quickly as possible. Once you've caught your breath, jog again until you feel you've had enough. At that point, walk again. Repeat this series of walking and jogging intervals for 30 minutes. If you stick with this method, you'll find over time that you can increase the jogging intervals and decrease the walking intervals until you can jog for the entire 30 minutes. Plan your route to make it as scenic as possible to help you enjoy your run.
Cool-down	Standing hamstring and calf stretch (30-40 sec each leg); walking quad stretch (30-40 sec each leg); lying knee to chest (30-40 sec each leg); and upper-back reach stretch (30-40 sec)

Intermediate Running Fusion Workout

If you already have some running experience, the intermediate running fusion workout in figure 14.8 will help you move to higher levels of running and further increase your endurance and cardiorespiratory fitness.

FIGURE 14.8   Intermediate Running Fusion Workout

Warm-up	Perform the basic warm-up, intermediate warm-up or advanced warm-up from round 5.
Flexibility exercises	*Perform 2-3 exercises for 1 minute each:* Bend and flex, hamstring and calf stretch, hip flexion with rotation, hip rotation, inward shoulder stretch, lateral lunge, lunge with rotation, lying knee to chest, outward shoulder stretch, plank with rotational reach, single-leg wall reach, spiderman climb, toe reach and touch, or total-body training stretch

Main session	Jab and cross (5 sets of 10 jabs with 8-10 sec rests between sets; 5 sets of 10 crosses with 8-10 sec rests between sets)	Jab-cross combination (5 sets with 8-10 sec rests between sets)	2-2-2-2 pattern: 2 forward shuffles, 1 jab-cross, 2 backward shuffles, 1 jab-cross, 2 left shuffles, 1 jab-cross, 2 right shuffles, 1 jab-cross (three 2 min rounds with 45 sec rests between rounds) (see round 6)

Intermediate running routine (30 min)	This routine incorporates fartlek training. *Fartlek* is a Swedish term that means 'speed play' and refers to a form of interval training that enhances both speed and endurance. A simple way to include fartlek training into your running is to use markers such as streetlights. Run at a steady pace towards a predetermined street light in the distance; when you reach it, increase your pace. Your breathing shouldn't be totally out of control, but it is completely normal if it gets heavier; this signals that your cardiorespiratory system is working harder. Once you've reached your second landmark (e.g., the next street light), slow your pace to below your normal running pace and stay at that pace until you've fully recovered and your breathing has returned to normal. Repeat these intervals for 30 minutes.
Cool-down	Standing hamstring and calf stretch (30-40 sec each leg); walking quad stretch (30-40 sec each leg); lying knee to chest (30-40 sec each leg); and upper-back reach stretch (30-40 sec)

Advanced Running Fusion Workout

If you are already an experienced runner (e.g., you run at least a 30-minute route three times per week or more) and you find the basic and intermediate running fusion workouts too easy, try this advanced workout in figure 14.9.

FIGURE 14.9 Advanced Running Fusion Workout

Warm-up	Perform the basic warm-up, intermediate warm-up or advanced warm-up from round 5.		
Flexibility exercises	*Perform 2-3 exercises for 1 minute each:* Bend and flex, hamstring and calf stretch, hip flexion with rotation, hip rotation, inward shoulder stretch, lateral lunge, lunge with rotation, lying knee to chest, outward shoulder stretch, plank with rotational reach, single-leg wall reach, spiderman climb, toe reach and touch, or total-body training stretch		
Main session	Jab and cross (5 sets of 10 jabs with 8-10 sec rests between sets; 5 sets of 10 crosses with 8-10 sec rests between sets)	Jab-cross combination (5 sets with 8-10 sec rests between sets)	2-2-2-2 pattern: 2 forward shuffles, 1 jab-cross, 2 backward shuffles, 1 jab-cross, 2 left shuffles, 1 jab-cross, 2 right shuffles, 1 jab-cross (three 2 min rounds with 45 sec rests between rounds) (see round 6)
Advanced running routine (30 min)	With the advanced running routine, you get out in the fresh air to further boost your metabolic fire with a hill sprint workout of 25 metres × 4 (100 m for each sprint). Starting at the bottom of the hill, fix on a point that is about 25 metres away and sprint towards it. When you hit that point, turn around and return to the starting point at a steady jog. On reaching the starting point, fix your focus on the 25-metre point and repeat the sprint; do this four times with two-minute rest periods between sprints (that's 400 m in total). Before you begin your hills sprints, take some time to visualise what you will achieve. See yourself powerfully sprinting towards the top of the hill, feel the energy pulsing in your body as the wind rushes past your head. Make the picture as bright and clear as possible. Finish with a steady jog to allow your body to recover and reduce your blood lactate level. As you do, reflect on what you have achieved during the session and how much closer you are to achieving your fitness goals. And don't forget to do your stretches at the end of every workout.		
Cool-down	Standing hamstring and calf stretch (30-40 sec each leg); walking quad stretch (30-40 sec each leg); lying knee to chest (30-40 sec each leg); and upper-back reach stretch (30-40 sec)		

This is it! You have been through an amazing journey packed with workouts that will have a huge impact on your fitness, health and overall well-being. This round provided the final suggestion: to integrate fun exercise routines into your workouts and your life. Keep up the good work, and whenever you need some inspiration, pick up this book again and choose the workout that suits you.

About the Authors

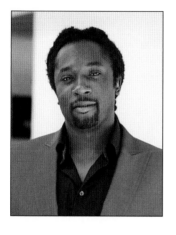

Martin McKenzie is a mind and movement specialist, celebrity trainer, boxing consultant and top performance and transformational coach. He is also the founder of Fight Fit Training and Development Ltd., a unique company delivering high-energy boxing for fitness classes and accredited courses, workshops and franchises for fitness professionals. The workouts featured in this book are part of the Fight Fit training systems and have been enjoyed by thousands worldwide. McKenzie's mind–body training system takes the unique approach of engaging the mind first to produce specific results in the body, such as increased speed, power and accuracy and healthy accelerated weight loss. McKenzie's methods are highly sought after by top celebrities, elite athletes and people who want to get to the top of their game while maintaining the highest level of mind–body fitness.

McKenzie's methods have saved boxing champions and mixed martial artists effort and injuries by giving them that vital competitive edge in a shorter time. He has spent many years working with the UK's most exclusive clubs to enhance their approach to overall fitness and health. McKenzie has also worked with the UK government and health ministers to tackle the global epidemic of obesity.

Because of the success of his methodologies, McKenzie creates strategies and interventions for various Forbes 500 companies and runs lectures and training courses for organisations worldwide.

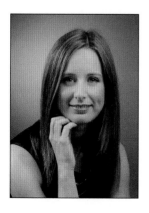

Stefanie Kirchner is a respected holistic health practitioner, lifestyle coach and nutrition therapist and runs a private practise at the prestigious Harley Street in London. She designs unique lifestyle and diet programmes for her clients, including top athletes and celebrities. Kirchner also consults charitable organisations on their development of international food campaigns and the promotion of a healthy lifestyle. For more information on Kirchner's services, visit www.nutritionbystefanie.com.

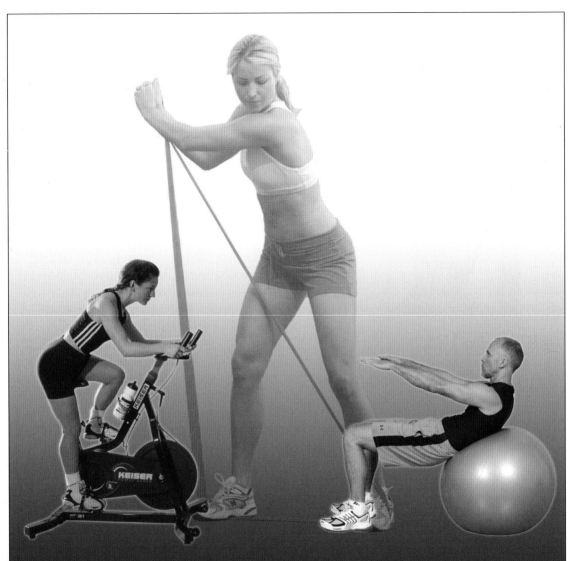